NEUROLOGIC EXAMINATION

ROBERT J. SCHWARTZMAN, MD

ISBN Hardback: 978-1-7345967-0-0
ISBN Softback: 978-1-7345967-3-1
ISBN eBook: 978-1-7345967-2-4
Library of Congress Control Number: 2020903413
DOI: 10.37913/NE.2020903413.0

Neurologic Examination is an illustrated guide for all aspects of the neurologic exam. This book is designed to help medical personnel make a diagnosis with the patient's history and physical examination; it leads the physician to the correct localization of a lesion utilizing simple bedside tests. The only tools employed are a reflex hammer and a pin. The illustrations and technique descriptions guide the practitioner through subtle but important details and distinctions, which include the observation of gait, the use of drifts, arm roll, and parietal copy.

1. Motor Exam   2. Cranial Nerves   3. Sensory Exam   4. Cerebellar Exam
5. Neurological Exam   6. Coordination   7. Reflexes   8. Mental Status
9. Patient History   10. Abnormal Sensation

I Schwartzman, Robert J. MD   II Neurologic Examination

Neurologic Examination may be purchased at special quantity discounts for colleges, universities, or educational purposes for medical schools, physician offices, research, or educational purposes.
For more information, contact Kirsten Erwin: rjsmedicalpress@gmail.com.

Cover and Interior Layout: Megan Leid
Publishing Consultant: Mel Cohen inspiredauthorspress@gmail.com
Contact: Kirsten Erwin at rjsmedicalpress@gmail.com for reprints of specific chapters or the entire book, and Rights or Licensing Agreements
Publisher: RJS Medical Press LLC
Website: www.rjsmedicalpress.com
Printed in the United States of America

Contents

Foreword to *Neurologic Examination*

I had the good fortune to do my residency training under Dr. Schwartz-man and even became his chief resident. He would make a point of spending some extra time after work with his chiefs because they have such a great deal of responsibility. This informal setting provided an opportunity to learn from the man who is both a great teacher and a good human being. We would review the past week's cases; he would offer guidance regarding the management of the residents and medical students. It was a time where I was taught how to be both a good physician and a person who makes (or helps families make) difficult decisions for another human being who is someone's parent, sibling, or child.

Years later, becoming the chair of the same neurology department left me with some big shoes to fill. For nearly two decades, Dr. Schwartzman has been my mentor: from my residency to my chairmanship.

This book has so much knowledge that it can serve everyone from the novice to the well-seasoned neurologist. The novice will gain the ability to master and interpret the examination, while well-seasoned specialists will find a treasure trove of nuances in the examination's interpretation. The book is very well organized, and that is what makes it so easy to use as a reference. I cannot imagine a better person to describe and teach a thorough neurological examination as well as the interpretation from its findings as Dr. Robert Schwartzman.

A good number of years have passed since completing a neurology residency with Dr. Schwartzman; still, every time I meet with my former colleagues, at some point, our conversation always drifts to remembering our days with him. We still reminisce about his morning reports and the Grand Rounds, where he led a live patient presentation examination every Friday. That is where we all learned the importance and nuances of the neurological examination. I think all of his trainees would agree that there was no better person to teach it than Dr. Robert Schwartzman.

We were all very fortunate to have had him as our teacher and mentor; there were many times when the thought of how to preserve this knowledge would cross my mind. Knowing that Dr. Schwartzman has written a detailed, illustrated book about the neurological examination makes me grateful that this knowledge will not be lost and will be available to future generations. This book will always be relevant since the thorough evaluation of a patient with neurological disorders remains very dependent on a reliable and precise examination.

Following in the steps of Dr. Schwartzman is not an easy task. For me, and for all of his trainees (and there are a lot of us out there), this book serves as a testament to our great teacher. This knowledge is now available for others to use.

Enjoy and learn,
G. Peter Gliebus, MD, FAAN
Academic Chairman of Neurology, Drexel University College of Medicine
Director of Cognitive Disorders Center, Global Neurosciences Institute,
Philadelphia, PA
Author of *Progressive Cognitive Impairment and Its Neuropathologic Correlates*

Endorsements

"This book teaches you the finesse and subtlety of a neurological examination. It is a part of my clinical practice and has never failed me to help my patients. The skillset you acquire with practicing the 'RJS way' makes one an unbeatable neurologist!"

Rohini Bhole, MD
Assistant Professor
Department of Neurology
University of Tennessee Health Science Center
Memphis TN 38163

"For everyone who is trying to master the neurological examination: this book is very useful to all—from medical students to practicing neurologists. It should be a part of the neurology training curriculum."

G. Peter Gliebus, MD
Director, Cognitive Disorders Center
Global Neurosciences Institute
Philadelphia, PA

"Dr. Schwartzman's *Neurologic Examination* is the foundation of my training in neurology. Not only does it provide the basics of the neurological exam but provides in-depth instruction in the exam of the cervical plexus, brachial plexus, and the chronic pain (Complex Regional Pain Syndrome) patient."

Lara Edinger, DO
Edinger Pain Management
10921 Wilshire Blvd., Suite 1109
Los Angeles, CA, 90024

"*Neurologic Examination* is a comprehensive volume by a master clinician on the topic. It is a lucid description of intricacies of neurologic examination with pithy discussions of interpretation and pathophysiology of the findings. It is a great resource for students, trainees and seasoned neurologists alike. The volume incorporates up to date neuroscience finding while preserving the methodology of classic and time-tested approach to the neurologic examination. Both neurologist and primary care clinicians would benefit and learn from the new edition of *Neurologic Examination*."

S. Ausim Azizi, MD PhD
Director of Neurology
Global Neuroscience Institute
Professor of Neurology (Adj.)
Temple University School of Medicine
Philadelphia, PA

"To find a comprehensive neurology book is always nice. To discover a neurology book that is an encyclopedia and yet easy to follow is indeed a good fortune... While I didn't have the opportunity to learn directly from Dr. Schwartzman, I find the illustrations and detailed descriptions to be a comprehensive guide to his wisdom. The sheer amount of knowledge contained in the *Neurologic Examination* book makes it a powerful tool to learn and master the neurologic examination. It is a concise and a must-have textbook for both the budding and advanced neurologists. This book is elegant; I will only replace it with a newer edition of itself!"

Mustafa J. Zahmak, MD, MPH
Neurooncology fellow, Yale University
New Haven, CT

"Reading *Neurologic Examination* is like rounding with Dr. Schwartzman again, one of the most skilled clinical neurologists of modern times. It is a refresher and source of fond memories for the hundreds of trainees who were fortunate enough to have him as a teacher and a treasure trove of clinical tricks and secrets for those who were not. Take it all in – and then live it for the rest of your career!"

Joachim M. Baehring, MD, DSc
Professor, Departments of Neurology and Neurosurgery
Vice-Chair, Clinical Affairs, Department of Neurology
Yale School of Medicine
Associate Chief of Neurology, Yale, New Haven Hospital, New Haven, CT

Preface

I am deeply honored to have the opportunity to join my illustrious predecessors in preparing this first edition of Neurologic Examination, which follows very closely the style of the sixth edition of Dr. Bickerstaff's Neurological Examination in Clinical Practice. I have kept to its major organizational pattern but have tried to add a small amount of physiology and anatomy to help the practitioner in understanding the neurologic signs that he has elicited. I have expanded the differential diagnoses to include newly described entities. It is my hope that some of the new examination techniques illustrated will garner the diagnosis on clinical grounds prior to evaluation by modern imaging techniques. The old formula honed to a cutting edge by all of the great British neurologists still holds, localization first and then differential diagnosis.

A discussion of ancillary components of the clinical examination such as electroencephalography (EEG), electromyography (EMG) and magnetic resonance imaging (MRI) techniques are beyond the scope of this book and have been omitted.

Hopefully, the book will guide students and residents in the neurologic sciences to an organized approach to their neurologically ill patient.

Grateful thanks are due to Kelly Malloy, O.D. (Pennsylvania College of Optometry) for the optic nerve photographs, to my two models Marielle Perreault and Kirsten Erwin; Senior Editor, Stuart Taylor and Assistant Development Editor, Rob Blundell. Stuart Taylor was particularly encouraging during a period of useful criticism by reviewers. Rob Blundell successfully guided the book through production. Special thanks to Sheila Urban who patiently waded through my horrible handwriting to type the manuscript; Dr. John Grothusen who photographed the new illustrations; my administrators Janet McCracken and Barbara Erwins-Romm who helped prevent me from getting everything mixed up and anonymous appreciation to all of the students, residents and colleagues who helped me to develop the neurologic examination that is presented.

This book is affectionately dedicated to the ones I love, my wife Denise and our children, Jane, Nancy and David.

Robert J. Schwartzman, MD
Philadelphia, 2006

1: The History

Neurology remains the specialty in medicine that still requires a good history and examination to diagnose a puzzle. It is ultimately logical and the approach leads the physician to localize the lesion to a part of the neuraxis and then develop a differential diagnosis based on this localization. The imaging tools are now superb, but must be applied correctly and their limitations understood. There is no imaging device that can diagnose a migraine headache. A purist might argue that a spreading depression of Leão might accomplish this with positron emission tomography (PET), but unfortunately other pathologies can cause the same physiology. Magnetic resonance imaging (MRI) does not evaluate bones well because a signal cannot be generated from a calcium lattice (no free H^+). A negative MRI of the spine in a patient with clear L5–S1 symptomatology, a weak extensor hallucis longus muscle and a depressed ankle jerk has overwhelming evidence of L5, S1 pathology. An older patient has bone disease of the spine rather than disk disease. This is not understood by most who hold the MRI as the gold standard for diagnosis of spinal problems. Complicated spine problems require a myelogram with contrast to evaluate the relationship of the nerve root to the facet, pedicle and exit foramina. These studies may be negative, but the patient still complains of severe L5–S1 pain. Recent information suggests that inflammatory cytokines released at an area of injury may directly stimulate C and A-delta pain fibers. If all imaging studies are negative as well as the electromyogram (EMG), but the history and the neurologic examination is positive, the examiner believes the patient and does the best that can be done to relieve the pain.

A productive way to look at modern neurology is that the history gives the diagnosis, the neurologic examination proves it and modern imaging and laboratory tests guide the treatment and predict the prognosis.

Localization by chief complaint

An accurate chief complaint must be given by the patient if possible. Specific pathologies cause very specific chief complaints although the patient may have severe simultaneous deficits. These cannot be summarized as the examiner loses the flavor of the core of the process.

Inability to express oneself with intact understanding is almost always a problem in Broca's area (44), the supplementary motor cortex or, rarely, the thalamus. Inability to understand the spoken word, with sudden onset and no other symptomatology in a patient with atrial fibrillation almost

1

always indicates an embolus to the inferior division of the middle cerebral artery that involves the superior temporal gyrus (Broadman's area 21, 22) or Wernicke's area.

A patient with severe short-term memory loss, retained social graces and some parietal symptomatology has Alzheimer's disease until proven otherwise. A patient who appears demented, but fluctuates in disease severity and has visual hallucinations most often has diffuse Lewy body disease.

Behavioral neurology is based on deficits in distributed loops, which is how nuclei of the brain interact one with the other. This physiology is the basis for the chief complaint. If the caregiver states that their charge seems to be able to see, but cannot reach objects, the examiner suspects a vascular or mass lesion that interrupts posterior parietal areas that integrate visual information with hand function (Balint's syndrome).

Any chief complaint that incorporates an agnosia, an inability to recognize an object, sound or tactile sensation with intact primary visual, auditory and somesthetic primary modality function, suggests a cortical process. Apraxias, in which a patient has normal strength, coordination and sensory abilities but cannot perform specific one command or sequential command motor acts, suggests cortical pathology. The chief complaint of these patients, often related by the caregiver, is, "Mr. Jones can no longer tie his shoes or use the telephone."

Knowledge of personal spaces that one can touch, and extrapersonal space, is biased toward the right parietal lobe. Patients with posterior right parietal lobe lesions ignore the left side of space. They frequently bump into objects on the left side of their personal space because they are unaware of it. These patients often are seen in the Emergency Room as a result of car accidents. The patient is frequently unaware of the deficit.

Each component of the cortex has anatomy and physiology that leads to a specific chief complaint.

The speed of development of the chief complaint gives insight into localization and pathologic process. If Mr. Jones's caregiver states that he is very rapidly losing intellectual function over a matter of weeks and has developed abnormal movements (myoclonus), the diagnosis is most likely prion disease of the classic Creutzfeldt–Jakob variety. A patient who is focused on a severe right parietal headache, particularly with standing and associated weakness of the left side, is an excellent candidate for a right-sided subdural or hemispheric brain tumor.

Seizures are particularly likely to announce their origin in the brain by their inscription, the initial area of discharge. A patient who states, prior to losing consciousness, that he or she smelled "rotting garbage" has a discharge from the uncus of the hippocampal gyrus. The examiner suspects seizures from the length of time the patient lost consciousness and was not completely him or herself. Seizures cause a change of mental states for minutes to hours in most instances. A syncopal attack, whether vagovagal or vasodepressor, lasts seconds. A cardiac arrhythmia causes loss of consciousness for 30 seconds to 1 minute unless it results in death. A transient ischemic attack (TIA) of the posterior or anterior circulation usually does not cause loss of consciousness. Shaking or apparent clonus may occur with weakness of an extremity from a carotid TIA. A drop attack, most often from posterior circulation ischemia of the medial reticular formation or possibly the cerebral peduncle or medullary pyramidal tract, does not cause loss of consciousness in most instances. Patients appear stunned. In a TIA, the larger the embolic material (red from the heart), the larger and longer the ischemic deficit. Most TIAs are short, 30 seconds to 2 minutes, and the emboli material seen in retinal arteries is yellow (cholesterol) from an intra-arterial source. A patient's chief complaint of falling when arising in the morning on the way to the bathroom suggests a thrombosis of the right middle cerebral artery (MCA), which leaves him unaware of the left side. Thrombotic strokes occur in the morning (4–6 AM), whereas emboli and hypertensive hemorrhages occur during the day.

Falling as a major complaint is common in elderly patients. The examiner determines in which direction the patient falls. Falling backwards is common with all basal ganglia disease, but particularly progressive supranuclear palsy, normal pressure hydrocephalus and acquired hepato-lenticular degeneration. Falling to one side is indicative of cerebellar disease or contralateral hemispheric disease. A patient stating that he or she is "pushed" to a "side" or "driven" to a side often has vestibular disease. Recently, posterior thalamic hemorrhages have been shown to cause patients to push away from the lesioned side. This lesion causes a deficit in the patient's sense of where their body is in relation to the vertical plane (an internal compass now known as the subjective visual vertical or SVV). These patients are knows as "pushers." Falling or being "pushed" forward is disease of the utriculus and sacculus.

The most prominent complaint of patients with basal ganglia disease is often difficulty with walking. The problem is frequently one of gait ignition failure. A similar gait difficulty occurs with normal pressure hydrocephalus (NPH) but is associated with cognitive decline and precipitates micturition. The patient with Parkinson's disease, in addition to the major difficulty with gait, complains of drooling, stiffness, tremor and fatigue. While taking this history, the examiner notes a serpentine stare, failure to blink (less than 14 times/minute) and a paucity of spontaneous movements. The patient will give the major complaint in a low voice.

If tremor is the major concern of the patient, the examiner can immediately and logically separate the process as one emanating from the basal ganglia or the cerebellum and its connections. In general, the tremor occurs at rest or with intention. A pill rolling tremor at rest (4–7, H2) with flexion of the metacarpophalangeal joint indicates Parkinson's disease. Tremors that occur with intention emanate from the cerebellum or its connections. A side-to-side tremor is strong evidence of an essential cerebellar tremor. An intention tremor with major oscillations is a cerebellar outflow or a rubral tremor. If it occurs in a young patient, the usual diagnosis is multiple sclerosis (MS). If it appears after head trauma, the midbrain (areas close to the red nucleus) is damaged. Rarely, movement disorder indicates choreoathetosis, myoclonus or dystonia.

Most patients with primary brainstem lesions complain of diplopia, dysphagia or dysarthria. Oscillopsia, in which objects in the environment are "jumping up or down" or otherwise moving, occurs with acute nystagmus. If the examiner notes severe nystagmus but the patient does not complain of oscillopsia, it has been compensated and is of long duration.

The outstanding complaint of patients with cerebellar disease is being "off balance" or "walking like a drunk." These patients also complain of poor handwriting that is too large, sloppy and not legible. They have major difficulty with fine movements such as drinking coffee or buttoning a shirt. If dysarthria is prominent, a spinocerebellar degeneration is suspected (degeneration of the left paravermian zone). Alcoholic cerebellar degeneration primarily affects the anterior lobules of the vermis and gait is more affected than the arm, speech or eyes (minimal nystagmus). Pes cavus is frequently seen with hereditary cerebellar degeneration and dysarthria. Vestibular disease patients often complain of being lightheaded or, as noted earlier, may feel as if they are being pushed.

Intrinsic or extrinsic spinal cord disease is often announced by the feeling of a tight band around the chest. This may at times be painful and unilateral. Patients feel that their legs are heavy after they walk a few blocks. They usually are unaware that bladder, bowel and coordination are affected. If bilateral optic neuritis and concomitant spinal cord involvement occurs, this is most often Devic's disease, a variant of MS. The usual band is felt at T1–T4 but this is often a dropped level because of cervical cord inflammation that affects the lamination of the spinothalamic tract. If the band is painful at T1–T4, cardiac disease is often suspected. An electrocardiogram (ECG) is certainly justified, but weak legs certainly suggest a spinal cord origin of the constrictive band sensation.

Fatigue as a major component of a neurologic symptom complex is characteristic of demyelinating, chronic fatigue syndrome and basal ganglia disease. It is a major and often the chief complaint of patients with depression, cancer, anemia, thyroid, congestive heart failure and Addison's disease. If the patient with severe fatigue also complains of Lhermitte's sign (paresthesias of the hands and arms with neck flexion) and is 20–40 years of age, the most likely diagnosis is MS.

The chief complaint of patients with diseases of the peripheral nervous system is equally as helpful as those who have disease of the central nervous system (CNS) in identifying whether the problem is at a root, plexus, neuromuscular junction or muscle level. The specific, sensory, chief complaint of the patient with a peripheral neuropathy identifies the size of the affected fibers which, when coupled with the pattern, evolution and associated features of the process, allow the examiner to categorize the neuropathy immediately.

Burning feet suggests that C fibers (1 μm unmyelinated) are spontaneously firing. If the strength and reflexes are relatively preserved, the patient has a small fiber neuropathy. The usual causes are diabetes, alcohol or human immunodeficiency virus (HIV). Unusual causes are Sjögren's syndrome, an autoimmune or specific antigens of the peripheral nerve. Numbness and slight weakness of the lower extremities suggests a dying back or metabolic neuropathy. This impression is further enhanced if the patient states that when the numbness reached the knees he or she started to lose sensation in the fingers. A similar process obtains with the intercostal nerves whose distal-most fibers innervate the anterior chest wall. This causes a "shield pattern" of sensory loss. The size of fibers that are involved in many metabolic dying back neuropathies are 8–10 μm in diameter. They mediate light touch, tap, pressure and motor function. In distinction to patients with a metabolic or dying back neuropathy, patients who complain of minimal numbness but extreme weakness of the legs that is progressing have Guillain–Barré syndrome. In this instance, large neurons of the dorsal root ganglia as well as an alpha fiber (12–22 μm) are affected.

Asymmetric weakness initially striking the upper rather than the lower extremities suggests an autoimmune large fiber neuropathy, with the GM1 epitope as the antigenic stimulus. A small fiber neuropathy is suggested by coldness of the hands (involvement of 1 μm sympathetic fibers that innervate blood vessels) and low blood pressure with intact strength and reflexes.

Lancinating pain is characteristic of root disease and is carried by A-delta (1–4 μm) thinly myelinated fibers. They are often the first impinged upon by an extruded disk that compresses the lateral component of the dorsal root entry zone as it pierces the dura on its way to the dorsal horn of the spinal cord. If this pain radiates into the buttock, lateral thigh and dorsum of the foot to the great toe, the L5 root is the culprit. In general, upper extremity radicular disease radiates to the shoulder, spinous processes and, rarely, to the fingers. Lower extremity radicular pain characteristically radiates to the toe and foot as well as back and buttock. Disturbing to both patient and examiner is the fact that radicular pain is often "striplike" in character. One day it is lateral thigh, the next, back and buttock, and the following week the top of the foot and great toe. It rarely covers the entire distribution of the root. As the more medial fibers of the dorsal root entry zone are compressed, sensations switch from lancinating to paresthetic and then to numbness. Patients may also complain of the blended sensations of burning, numbness and cold lancinating pain.

In the lower extremity, the examiner is able to utilize quality of sensation distribution of sensory abnormality and exacerbating and relieving factors to deduce both physiology and pathology. A patient with spinal stenosis will state that he or she can only walk a block or so and then has to rest because his or her legs are heavy and painful. The most pain is often in the calves and is usually described as a cramp, tightness or a "charley horse." These are neurogenic cramps from activation of deep muscle A-delta pain afferents. A patient with vascular insufficiency of the iliac arteries complains of tightness and a burning sensation in the calves, thighs and buttocks. The burning sensation is from activation of C fibers due to lactic

5

acidosis. Someone with Buerger's disease has intermittent claudication of the inner side of the foot. Walking that causes intermittent claudication of vision indicates Takayasu's disease (pulseless disease of young women).

In general, the chief complaint of patients who suffer brachial plexus disease is pain. The usual cause is a traction injury such as a motor vehicle accident or fall on the outstretched upper extremity. The radiations are to the trapezius ridge and medical scapular border (upper trunk) as well as the 4th and 5th fingers (lower trunk). The sympathetic system is frequently activated abnormally and patients often gradually develop burning pain in a regional distribution (chronic regional pain syndrome). Unless there is actual avulsion of the roots such as occurs with severe trauma (motorcycle accident), weakness and wasting are less than that noted with radicular disease. As noted earlier, root disease in the upper extremity rarely reaches the hand. C4 radiates along the trapezius ridge, C5 to the cap of the shoulder and C6 to the lateral forearm and, rarely, to the thumb and index fingers. Thus, in general, a patient with pain or paresthesias that radiate into the hand have median or ulnar neuropathy or plexus disease.

Patients with the most common neuromuscular junction disease, myasthenia gravis, complain most commonly of cranial nerve dysfunction such as ptosis or diplopia and secondarily fatigue and weakness with exercise. The other neuromuscular junction illnesses are uncommon and have specific seminal symptoms. A patient with small cell cancer of the lung who has the paraneoplastic antibody induced Lambert–Eaton syndrome has a dry mouth and "load in the pants" gait. The patient has developed antibodies to the L-type calcium channels on the terminal twigs of the muscle fibers at the neuromuscular junction as well as to the salivary glands. These patients get stronger rather than weaker with exercise, as opposed to those with myasthenia gravis. Patients with botulism often present first with nausea and vomiting, ptosis and pupillary dilation in addition to pharyngeal and generalized weakness. On the other hand, tetanus strikes the masseter early and is noted for trismus, the patient reporting that he or she cannot open their mouth fully. Many patients with tetanus in the USA are intravenous drug abusers and come to the hospital late with severe stimulus-sensitive myoclonus.

Most muscle disease affects proximal muscle groups. Patients present with difficulty in getting out of a chair, holding their arms over their head or, rarely, with sore muscles. Patients with metabolic muscle disease present with cramps and, at times, myoglobinuria. After age 50, inclusion body myopathy should be suspected with acquired proximal myopathy, particularly if the forearm flexor muscles are involved.

In summary, each component of the neuraxis will generate a patient's chief complaint. This directs the examiner's attention to the relevant component of the neuraxis that has to be explored. It is surprisingly common to have patients describe their problems with the exact same words. Thus, each patient teaches the examiner.

The age of the patient is extremely important in determining a diagnosis as certain diseases occur at specific ages, which limits the differential diagnosis. In a young person, loss of consciousness for a few minutes is more likely to be a seizure than a cardiac arrhythmia. Double vision in a 20-year-old is more likely to be myasthenia gravis than brainstem vascular disease. A cerebellar tumor prior to age 12 will most likely be a medulloblastoma. A glioma, astrocytoma or ependymoma is more common at 15–20 years of age. If benign and lateral in a middle-aged man, it is likely to be a hemangioblastoma. A cerebellar lesion that occurs between the ages of 40 and 60 years will most often be a metastasis.

Clarifying the symptoms

What is important to the patient and the neurology resident may not be particularly relevant. Always listen carefully to the patient's symptoms and then use positive and negative questions to clarify the issue. In any pain problem, the examiner must identify:
1 the mode of onset;
2 the quality and severity of the pain;
3 its radiations;
4 relieving and exacerbating factors;
5 associated signs and symptoms.
It is rare that the diagnosis will be missed if this plan is followed. Dizziness is hard to clarify with anyone. Patients describe dizziness as lightheadedness, presyncope or a rotary feeling. Usually, the examiner can tease out if the environment seems to be moving or the patient (subjective vs. objective) and, most importantly, if there are any other associated signs or symptoms such as weakness, numbness or difficulty swallowing. If the symptom is just related to dizziness and there are no associated signs and symptoms, overwhelmingly the cause is peripheral (i.e., from the nerve or the labyrinth). Weakness, cranial nerve involvement and sensory loss make it a brainstem problem. Rarely, dizziness associated with weakness can be in the carotid rather than posterior circulation territory (the intraparietal sulcus receives vestibular input). The cortex receives all sensory projections and blends them into a perception.

Exact radiations of pain or distributions of sensory loss are very important. Numbness around both sides of the mouth is often ischemia of descending tracts of the sensory component of the fifth nerve. At the corner of the mouth and in association with the thumb and index finger, a cheiro-oral pattern is often seen with migraine. A tongue that is numb on one side alone is brainstem ischemia, while bilateral intra-oral numbness is of thalamic origin.

Each process that the patient suffers has a characteristic pattern, which is rarely psychiatric in origin. Patients do not like or pay doctors; they come to you because they are sick.

Mode of onset and progression

Apoplectic deficits in neurologic patients are vascular or seizures. A patient who has a sudden overwhelming headache and then collapses with no focal signs has a subarachnoid hemorrhage. A middle-aged plethoric hypertensive male who collapses with a flaccid hemiparesis has a deep basal ganglionic hemorrhage. The patient who, while at the dinner table, is suddenly stunned and cannot speak has suffered an embolus. If the patient has atrial fibrillation, the embolus will go to the inferior division of the middle cerebral artery and affect Wernicke's area and he or she may speak incessantly, but incoherently.

Sudden loss of consciousness may be preceded by an aura such as smelling "something rotten." This is not an instantaneous perception and is most often a complex partial seizure. Dementia that is slowly progressive over 2 years and is predominantly associated with memory deficit is Alzheimer's disease. If the dementia is rapidly progressive over 3 months without weakness, it will be Creutzfeldt–Jakob disease. If focal signs are present, the most likely diagnosis is a frontal lobe mass lesion.

The examiner must determine if the process is steadily progressive, remittent or increasing in small steps. Relapsing and remitting processes suggest demyelinating disease if in the CNS or chronic inflammatory polyneuropathy (CIDP) if the peripheral nervous system is involved. An examiner may encounter episodic ataxia or a periodic paralysis that causes intermittent paralysis; both are channelopathies (abnormalities of components of calcium or sodium channels).

Chronologic sequence of events

This aspect of history taking will give very helpful information as to pathology. Neurologic function degenerates in the face of mass lesions, not only because of their destructive aspects in the local area of growth, but also by pressure or hydrocephalus. A patient with multi-infarct dementia will have a series of well-documented vascular events. Unfortunately, he or she may be unlucky enough to have concomitant Alzheimer's disease. Demyelinating disease gradually destroys much of the brain even in the face of normal-appearing white matter on MRI (MR spectroscopy demonstrates that it is not). Relapsing–remitting disease responds better than primary or secondary progressive disease to immunomodulation. All neurologic processes have a specific progression of loss of neurologic function which, if identified, leads to changes in therapy as well as corroboration of the initial diagnosis. A patient originally diagnosed with MS resulting from an isolated deficit, but without characteristic involvement of neural structures both in time and space, may have anything from Lyme's disease to metachromatic leukodystrophy. It is always wise to keep evaluating patients in light of the natural history of their diagnosis and response to therapy. Polymyositis that is not responding to therapy with immunosuppressants suggests an alternate diagnosis of inclusion body myositis. Similarly, a patient with an akinetic-rigid syndrome with many parkinsonian features, but a poor response to levodopa, should raise suspicion of multiple system atrophy as the correct diagnosis.

Value of negative information

Negative information is crucial in defining the fine points of the clinical history. It is similar to sculpture. Most of the history will outline the general category of disease, but the use of negative information sculpts the fine points. An episodic headache in a male that is severe, periodic, radiates to the eye at the same time during the night suggests cluster headache. If the examiner inquires about the trigeminal aspects of the headache, dilation of conjunctival vessels and tearing, it may be the entity of sudden neuralgi-form pain with conjunctival injection and tearing (SUNCT). Most will be cluster headaches as this is common whereas SUNCT is not. A strong family history of migraine in a patient who has fortification scotomata but without headache would suggest a migraine variant (acephalgic migraine). A negative family history will direct the examiner's attention to a possible lesion of the occipital lobe. Inquiring in regard to palinopsia (visual perseveration) and photopsia (spontaneous patterns) are helpful in placing a lesion in the occipital lobe or parietal-occipital junction, respectively. Nowhere in medicine is being a "splitter" (knowing the fine points between different entities) more important than being a "lumper" (knowing the general categories of disease). "Splitters" are smart and "lumpers" are lazy (a usual excuse for saying "Why do I have to know that?"). The reason to know the fine points of entities is to guide therapy and to be sure of the correct diagnosis. A patient with a paralyzed leg equal in extent to the paralysis of the face and arm but with a severe aphasia probably has a myocardial infarction (MI) (first division)/MCA occlusion rather than the precentral branch of the superior division of the MCA from the carotid artery. Intra-arterial urokinase is much more effective for possible therapy than intravenous tissue plasminogen activator (TPA) in this instance.

Excluding irrelevancies

This aspect of the history is very difficult for many physicians. The history guides one from A to B. Patients frequently are driven to recite all of the hospitalizations, physicians and missed diagnoses that have befallen them. It is best to take this mostly irrelevant, written information from the patient and place it on your side of the desk. Otherwise, a great deal of the history will be distraction as he or she fiddles with the papers instead of listening to your questions and trying to give a correct answer. Assure the patient that all of the information they have brought to the office will be examined later. It is best to have the patient directly in front of you as you write notes so they are not distracted. The physician who looks at MRI films while taking the history finds it difficult to form an independent judgment of the pathology and will no longer use his or her best judgment, skills and examination to form an opinion. Read the films after examining the patient. Unfortunately, this rarely occurs at any level of practice.

Interviewing relatives

The relatives, if present with the patient, can give valuable information as regards the family history, the events leading up to a loss of consciousness or the mode of onset of the neurologic event. If the patient is suspected of having a peripheral neuropathy or spastic paraparesis, looking at the relative's feet for pes cavus and testing their reflexes may be helpful.

2: Mental Status

Orientation

All normal people are oriented to time, place and person. Time may be the most subtle component of this orientation. Most people in the modern world are oriented to time within 15 minutes. Thus, every person should be oriented to no less than 15 minutes. If you are generous, you can give a patient to 30 minutes. Patients with dementia and parietal lobe lesions (particularly) the right side may be disoriented to place. Some parietal lobe patients have very bizarre ideas of place orientation. They believe that their present location is related or connected to another location. Right parietal lobe defects cause difficulties with intra- and extrapersonal space. In general, place disorientation is associated with severe organic brain disease. Inability to recognize one's person is seen with hallucination and delusions in the acute state and chronically with severe dementia.

Memory

The memory function of the brain is essential for modern human life. It is subdivided by behavioral neurologists into explicit, that which you can consciously recall, and implicit, that which is registered without conscious intent and can only be examined under special circumstances. Working memory describes that body of knowledge that can easily be recalled and used for everyday living.

For the neurologist, memory is divided into inscription, consolidation and long-term phases. Inscription is the first 30 seconds, which depends on reverberating circuits of the hippocampus and utilizes acetylcholine as the neurotransmitter. Consolidation is the time period between this 30 seconds and 3 minutes. During this period, messenger RNA is synthesized and the brain is on the way to long-term memory which depends on protein synthesis. It is during this 30 seconds to 3 minute interval that consolidation can be interrupted by intrusions. Long-term memory is stored throughout the brain and is lost by destruction of brain tissue. Classic short-term memory depends on the dorsal medial nucleus of the thalamus, the mamillary bodies, fornix and medial hippocampus. The dorsolateral prefrontal cortex retrieves memories. Forgetting may be the unfolding of proteins that have been synthesized.

Memory is tested by having the patient repeat three objects immediately and then 3 minutes later. The patient should be able to do this without difficulty. Long-term memory is tested by asking what he or she had for last night's dinner or events that have occurred of which he or she should be aware. Remember to ask the same three objects to every patient or you will forget them.

Complex partial seizures and transient global amnesia affect medial hippocampal structures. Seizures that discharge into the medial dorsal thalamic nucleus from the cortex may present with no prior aura. Patients with bilateral temporal lobe disease from herpes simplex encephalitis, trauma or pituitary irradiation will have deficient short-term memory. Alcohol damages both the mamillary bodies and dorsal medial thalamic nuclei, and interferes with recent memory as well as orientation in time and space to such a degree that patients frequently confabulate events to fill in memory gaps (Korsakoff's syndrome). This syndrome may also be duplicated by anterior communicating artery aneurysms or their surgical repair.

Judgment

Asking a patient to describe what they would do if they found a letter addressed to someone else is a good estimate of judgment. This question unveils some interesting psychiatric problems that might be missed without specific probing in this area.

Affect

Every intracranial process affects a patient's "feeling tone" or affect. The frontal lobe is usually divided functionally. The left side is responsible for execution and planning, speech and memory retrieved (dorsal lateral prefrontal cortex). The right frontal lobe is for behavior. Disinhibition of personal behavior, hygiene and sexual activity is seen with lesions in the right frontal lobe. Inappropriate jocularity or "witzelsucht" is common. This is the lobe most involved with emotional control and inhibition of the limbic system.

A temporal lobe personality is characterized by:
1 a schizoid affect;
2 hyperreligiosity;
3 hypergraphia; and
4 viscosity.

The latter trait is exemplified by "just one more question doctor." Lesions of both temporal lobes cause social disruption.

Parietal lobe dysfunction, particularly of the right side, causes a flat affect and an unemotional prosody of speech. Surprisingly, euphoria occurs with lesions of the inferior longitudinal fasciculus that connects the amygdala and hippocampus to parietal association areas. Thus, what we see can be matched with what has been seen before.

The caudate nucleus, particularly if damaged on the right side, causes restlessness and agitated behavior. The same is noted with lesions of the right temporal-parietal-occipital cortex and orbitofrontal cortex. Lesions of projections from the caudate nucleus to the frontal lobe are associated with "La Belle" indifference, often seen in multiple sclerosis (MS) patients.

Emotional incontinence, "laughing without mirth" and "crying without tears," is a major component of pseudobulbar palsy. This is most commonly seen with bilateral corticospinal damage from cerebral vascular disease and is also common in MS and head trauma. Patients with thalamic lesions have waxing and waning levels of consciousness, while those who suffer subfrontal disease have abulia. After taking the history, the physician should know if the "feeling tone" or affect of the patient is normal or which lobe of the brain he or she has been "talking to".

Intellectual function

Some feel that an excellent measure of intellectual function is the sum total of information amassed by the patient. By asking a patient of normal intelligence basic knowledge and to calculate, one gets a feeling for intellectual function. This, of course, is affected greatly by educational status.

Additions to the mental status

Visual praxis (Fig. 2.1)

Visual praxis tests the ability to copy a hand posture after seeing it for 2 seconds. The patient must see the hand (areas 7, 18, 19 of the occipital and

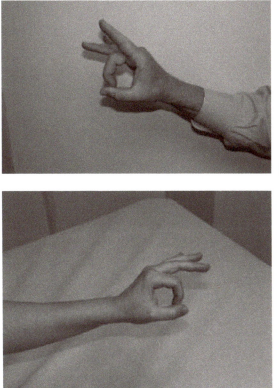

(a)

(b)

Fig. 2.1 Visual praxis. The patient is asked to copy the hand posture shown for 2 seconds. The hand is then removed. This type of deficit is seen in slightly demented patients.

parietal cortex), understand the command (Wernicke's area 22) and remember it (dorsal medial nucleus of the thalamus, formix, mamillary bodies and medial hippocampus) and have the ability to make an engram of movement (a motor program). A single engram is encoded in area 6 of the premotor cortex and activates area 4 of the motor cortex which initiates the motor program.

This simple maneuver tests visual and short-term memory as well as prefrontal and frontal lobe motor areas.

The four-part command (Fig. 2.2)

The four-part command requires the patient to take their right hand, touch their left ear, close their eyes and stick out their tongue. This requires that the patient know right from left (area 39, 40) of the left parietal cortex (LPC), cross the midline (area 39, 40 of the LPC), recognize body parts (right posterior parietal cortex), maintain their eyes closed (right parietal cortex; inability to do so is parietal impersistence) and the ability to perform all tasks without getting stuck on an earlier task (impersistence; left frontal cortex). The ability to remember all four commands tests short-term memory.

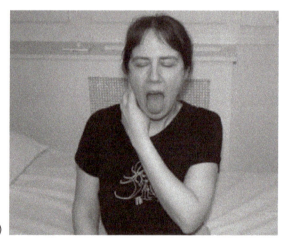

(a)

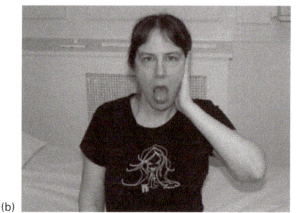

(b)

Fig. 2.2 The four-part command. (a) Normal response to four-part command. On command, the patient is able to follow the four commands: "Take your left hand, touch your right ear, close your eyes, and stick your tongue out." (b) The patient has failed to cross the midline and has been unable to keep her eyes closed.

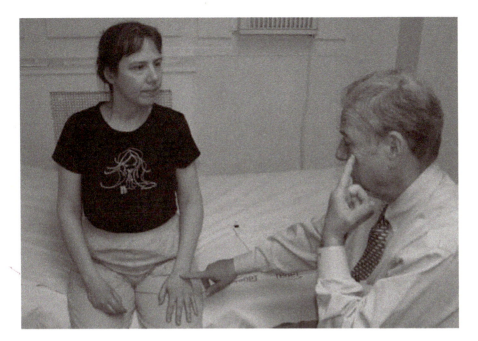

Fig. 2.3 The face–hand test. The patient is being asked, "Where did I touch you?"
If slightly confused (cortical level or demented), the patient reports, "On my face."

Thus, the four-part command tests Wernicke's area 22, the receptive speech area, major areas of the left parietal and frontal lobe, as well as short-term memory.

The face–hand test (Fig. 2.3)

If a patient has minimal cognitive dysfunction or the examiner feels there is a slight diminution of alertness, the examiner performs the face–hand test. The examiner, in the middle of a conversation, touches his or her face and the patient's hand. The examiner then asks the patient where he or she was touched and the patient will answer "my face." No normal patient makes this error.

3: Cranial Nerves

First cranial nerve

Very few things happen to the olfactory nerve (first). It should be tested carefully in head injury (where it is ripped from the cribriform plate), extra-parenchymal tumors of the base of the frontal lobe (meningioma of the olfactory groove) or intrinsic tumors of the nasal epithelium (neuroesthe-sioblastoma), vitamin B_{12} deficiency, Kallmann's syndrome (ovarian dys-genesis) and neurodegenerative disorders such as multiple system atrophy and Parkinson's disease.

Anatomy

Odorants excite neurons of the nasal mucosa, which project to the olfactory bulb, tract and roots (primarily the lateral root), which in turn project to the periamygdaloid and prepiriform cortex of the temporal lobe which then projects to the uncus and hippocarpal gyrus. Loss of olfactory sensation occurs primarily with bulb, tract and root lesions while olfactory hallucina-tions occur with medial temporal and uncal lesions. These are usually described as unpleasant smells such as burning rubber, rotten food or unde-sirable bad smells. Approximately 10% of reported smells are good, but usually are described as "too sweet." Olfactory auras are dramatically important in the diagnosis of medial temporal lobe epilepsy. Inferior frontal lobe gliomas may also present with bilateral anosmia.

Method of testing

Small bottles of coffee, almonds, chocolate and peppermint can be used. The test odor is placed under one nostril while the other is compressed. New scratch smell tests are now available. The patient is required to identify the odors. Patients who describe the odors as the same, but distorted and unpleasant, have paraosmia, often noted with Hencken's syndrome. This is a postviral phenomenon in which the nasal mucosa and the olfactory mucosa have been damaged. Paraosmia may occur because of incomplete olfactory recovery following head injury. Schizophrenia, depression and hysterical conversion syndromes have been described with these symp-toms. Rarely, patients with sarcoid, paraneoplastic syndromes, chronic meningitis and siderosis (iron deposition from recurrent intracranial bleed-ing) present with anosmia.

Second cranial nerve (Figs 3.1–3.4)

In general, in instances of visual loss or distortion, the most important point is if the dysfunction is in one or both eyes. If it can be localized to one eye, the pathology is in the retinal ganglion cells or the optic nerve. If it is clear that the loss is bilateral, the lesion must be in or posterior to the chiasm. Frequently, patients fail to recognize a nasal field deficit and describe their visual loss as only occurring in the eye with the temporal field deficit.

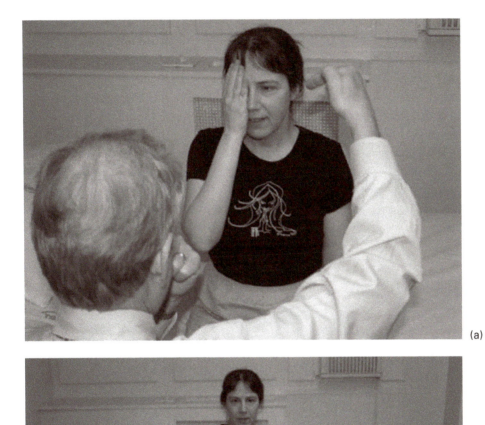

(a)

(b)

Fig. 3.1 (a) Monocular confrontation visual field testing. The patient is asked when the finger can be seen and when it has a flesh color to it (macular vision). (b) The patient is asked which hand is brighter and which hand moved when they are moved simultaneously. The examiner also notes gaze preference.

The advent of magnetic resonance imaging (MRI) has substantially altered visual field testing. The nuances of this test are passing into neurologic history. In general, MRI lesions should predict the visual field deficit. Visual field evaluation helps with following known lesions in demyelinating disease, retinal disease, glaucoma and macular disease.

Methods of testing

Confrontation (see Fig. 3.1)

The patient and examiner face each other at approximately 1 m. The patient covers one eye with a hand. The patient is asked to fix gaze between the examiner's eyes. The examiner notes to which side the patient looks if gaze is broken (patients invariably look into the normal hemifield). The examiner moves the index finger of the hand into each of the four quadrants from just outside the limits of his or her own field. It is often helpful to ask the patient not only when they can see the finger, but when they note it as flesh colored. A red object is better for this aspect of visual field testing as red desaturation (the color is not as bright as it should be or appears brown to the patient) is a marker of a lesion in the visual pathway. Graying of vision or color desaturation may be noted prior to a quantifiable visual field defect. If a defect is noted, it is better to test from blind areas

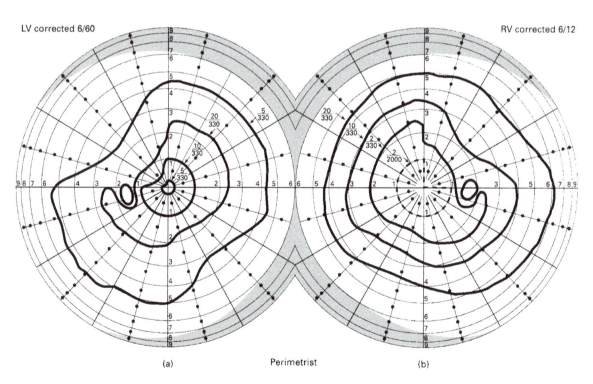

Fig. 3.2 Quantitative perimetry showing upper temporal quadrantic defects. (a) Charting a single small isoptre only (5/330) would give a wrong impression of merely a constricted field. (b) A large object would only show an almost normal field. By charting several different isoptres the clear-cut defect is uncovered.

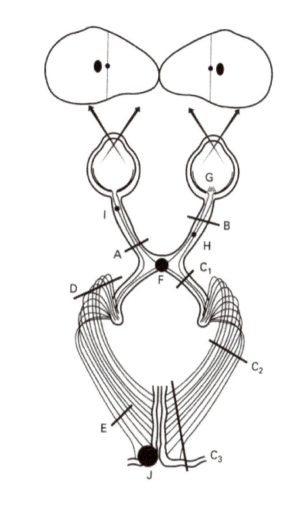

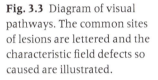

Fig. 3.3 Diagram of visual pathways. The common sites of lesions are lettered and the characteristic field defects so caused are illustrated.

to areas of preserved vision. Central vision is tested by utilizing a 5-mm white disk attached to a rod or long pin which detects enlarged blind spots or scotomata.

After each eye is tested separately, the examiner asks the patient to look (fix the vision) between the examiner's eyes. The examiner moves his or her hands separately in each quadrant and then simultaneously. If there is "perceptual rivalry" or inattention in one field and fingers are moved simultaneously, the patient will neglect or not perceive the finger subserving the damaged component of the visual pathway. This is the technique of double simultaneous stimulation (DSS). Rarely, a patient will not perceive an object in a damaged field that is stationary, but will see it instantly if it is moved (Riddoch's phenomenon). Quantitative perimetry is essential for accurate visual field testing (see Fig. 3.2). If objects of different sizes are used and larger objects are noted by the patient in the same sector of the field where smaller objects were missed, this suggests that the defect is partially caused by edema or pressure phenomena ("shading of a visual field"). An apparently constricted field demonstrated by small objects (2 mm) may actually hide a characteristic defect when 5- or 10-mm objects are utilized. Bjerrum screen (tangent screen) enlarges central meridians to 30° and is most helpful for measuring central scotomata and the blind spot.

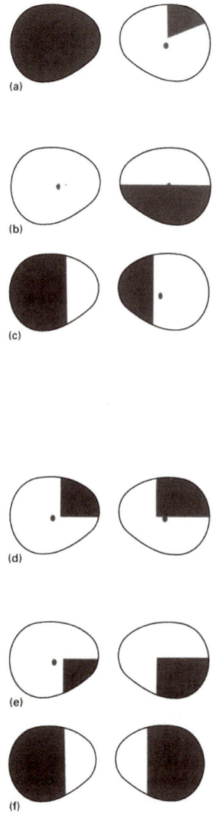

(a) **Total unilateral loss of vision**. A lesion of the optic nerve ("A" in Fig. 3.3)

Common causes: injuries, optic neuritis, optic nerve compression.

Involvement of nasal crossing fibers from the other eye will cause a contralateral upper temporal field defect (shaded area), usually with an ipsilateral scotoma rather than total blindness.

(b) **Altitudinous hemianopia**. A partial lesion of the blood supply to the optic nerve ("B" in Fig. 3.3).

Common causes: trauma, vascular accidents.

(c) **Homonymous hemianopia**. The most common major defect; caused by a lesion anywhere from optic tract to occipital cortex. In the *tract* it is usually complete, incongruous, without macular sparing ("C_1" in Fig. 3.3). In the *radiations* it is usually incomplete, congruous, with macular sparing ("C_2" in Fig. 3.3). In the *calcarine cortex* it is usually complete, congruous and with macular sparing, but may show associated scotomata ("C_3" in Fig. 3.3). Congruity and macular sparing are variable.

Common causes: vascular accidents, cerebral tumors, vascular anomalies, injuries.

(d) **Upper quadrantic homonymous defect**. Temporal lobe lesions involving the optic radiations where they sweep round the temporal horn of the lateral ventricle ("D" in Fig. 3.3). Less commonly in lower calcarine lesions; occasionally in partial tract lesions.

Common causes: cerebral tumors, vascular accidents, cerebral abscesses, injuries.

(e) **Lower quadrantic homonymous defect**. Lesions of the upper radiations or calcarine area ("E" in Fig. 3.3).

Common causes: vascular accidents, injuries, tumors.

(f) **Bitemporal hemianopia**. Lesions at the optic chiasma ("F" in Fig. 3.3).

Common causes: pituitary tumors, craniopharyngiomata, suprasellar meningiomas, midline aneurysms, hypothalamic neoplasms, gross IIIrd ventricular dilation, optic chiasmal gliomas.

Fig. 3.4 Examining the fundus.

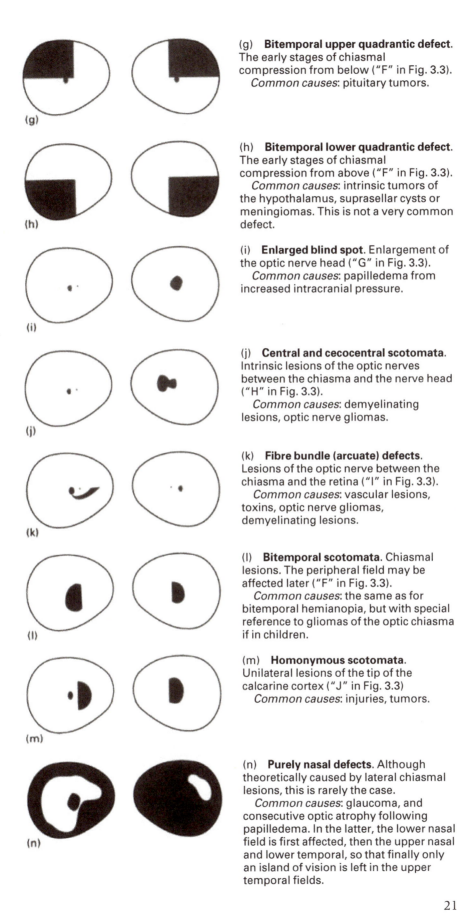

(g) Bitemporal upper quadrantic defect. The early stages of chiasmal compression from below ("F" in Fig. 3.3).
Common causes: pituitary tumors.

(h) Bitemporal lower quadrantic defect. The early stages of chiasmal compression from above ("F" in Fig. 3.3).
Common causes: intrinsic tumors of the hypothalamus, suprasellar cysts or meningiomas. This is not a very common defect.

(i) Enlarged blind spot. Enlargement of the optic nerve head ("G" in Fig. 3.3).
Common causes: papilledema from increased intracranial pressure.

(j) Central and cecocentral scotomata. Intrinsic lesions of the optic nerves between the chiasma and the nerve head ("H" in Fig. 3.3).
Common causes: demyelinating lesions, optic nerve gliomas.

(k) Fibre bundle (arcuate) defects. Lesions of the optic nerve between the chiasma and the retina ("I" in Fig. 3.3).
Common causes: vascular lesions, toxins, optic nerve gliomas, demyelinating lesions.

(l) Bitemporal scotomata. Chiasmal lesions. The peripheral field may be affected later ("F" in Fig. 3.3).
Common causes: the same as for bitemporal hemianopia, but with special reference to gliomas of the optic chiasma if in children.

(m) Homonymous scotomata. Unilateral lesions of the tip of the calcarine cortex ("J" in Fig. 3.3)
Common causes: injuries, tumors.

(n) Purely nasal defects. Although theoretically caused by lateral chiasmal lesions, this is rarely the case.
Common causes: glaucoma, and consecutive optic atrophy following papilledema. In the latter, the lower nasal field is first affected, then the upper nasal and lower temporal, so that finally only an island of vision is left in the upper temporal fields.

21

False positive defects

Bilateral defects of the upper or nasal fields may be caused by ptosis and large eyebrows or a large nose respectively. These are avoided by tilting or turning the patient's head. Patients with severe central scotomata cannot fix a central object. The patient is asked to hold the gaze on two objects at the edge of the scotomata while the remainder of the visual field is explored. Fixation can also be enhanced by enlarging the object of fixation. If visual acuity is good, a small concentrically constricted field is usually hysterical.

Funduscopic examination (Plate 1a, facing page 26)

The trick of a good fundus examination is resting the third finger on the patient's cheek to get as close to the pupil as possible. This takes practice. The light reflex is partially inhibited by decreasing the illumination of the room, while accommodation (which also constricts the pupil) is avoided by having the patient fix on a distant object.

Anatomy of the optic disk

The examiner must identify the disk and its components. Venous pulsations are noted in the center of the disk and not at its margins. This is a common mistake. As intracranial pressure increases it is transmitted to the eye via venous and cerebrospinal fluid pressure. If these combined pressures are greater than intraocular arterial pressure the veins will not collapse with the increment of arterial blood delivered to the rigid globe with each systole. Only if there is a wide systolic diastolic difference will venous pulsations be seen at the disk margin. This occurs with aortic insufficiency, severe hyperthyroidism or an arteriovenous fistula. The optic cup is in the center of the disk and has perforations from the optic nerve fibers, which are known as the lamina cribrosa. The examiner should note these in every patient as many changes in the disk both from pressure or systemic disease may be noted here. Deep nasalized cups are suggestive of glaucoma. An enlarged cup (excavated) and sharp disk margins suggests loss of optic nerve fibers. The color of the disk is important. It becomes erythematous in papilledema. Fat tortuous veins suggest polycythemia, Waldenström's macroglobulinemia or other hyperviscosity states. The nasal margins of the disk are usually blurred. The margins become indistinct with papilledema in a specific order: superior margin, inferior margin and temporal margin. The blood vessels of the retina are extremely helpful in diagnosis. Excessive elongation and tortuosity is characteristic of hypertension. A copper and silver wire appearance denotes severe atherosclerosis. "Commotio retina," an intense light streak, is seen with the severe vasospasm that occurs with acute head injury or Köhlmeier–Degos disease (arteritis with atrophic skin lesions). Arterial venous crossing points are accentuated in hypertension and often with collagen vascular disease. Hemorrhages from papilledema occur off the disk margin (slit hemorrhages); those from venous occlusion occur in the central retina and macula. A hemorrhage that moves with head position following a burst aneurysm is known as a preretinal or sub-hyaloid hemorrhage (Torsten's syndrome). This is important, as 20% of aneurysms are bilateral and the side of the hemorrhage is often the side of the aneurysm that burst.

The macula and fovea are examined by having the patient look directly at the light. The myriad of macular degenerative diseases are beyond the scope of neurologists. A great number of systemic diseases have ocular findings. The venous retinal hemorrhages of diabetes are well known as are the scattered hemorrhages of leukemia and other severe anemias. Patients with systemic lupus erythematosus may demonstrate cytoid bodies ("grain of rice") in the peripheral retina, while patients with severe renal disease show a combination of advanced atherosclerosis and accelerated hypertension leading to a macular star (edema outlining the nerve sheath layer).

All neurologists should be able to identify the branch point occlusion of a cholesterol embolus (Hollenhorst plaque). It is strikingly birefringent, yellow and often appears larger than the vessel it occludes. Platelet fibrin plaques from heparin-induced thrombocytopenia (HIT) are white and often multiple. Calcium, air and fat emboli can be seen in the retinal circulation.

The only way for the examiner to become proficient with the ophthalmoscope is to use it. Ask yourself if you have seen all components of the disk, the vessels and the macula. Recent experimental evidence points out the great similarity between the retinal and the cerebral circulations.

The disk (Plate 1b, 1c, 1d, facing page 26)

Pallor

An aspirin-white disk with sharp margins, often with the choroid exposed, denotes optic atrophy. This may be seen with destruction of the retina, optic nerve or anterior chiasm from injury, inflammation, compression, ischemia, mitochondrial disease (Leber's optic neuropathy), genetic or degenerative diseases.

It is rare to see long-standing papilledema in the West because of the advent of computed tomography (CT) and MRI. Optic pallor in this setting is often associated with fibrosis at the disk margin.

Temporal pallor is noted in any process that affects the maculopapillary bundle. It is seen frequently with the optic neuritis of multiple sclerosis. The examiner will note that this area of the disk is alabaster white and is bounded by a normal white grayish cup margin. The green light of the ophthalmoscope demonstrates the nerve fiber layer of the retina and delineates these fibers as they enter the disk. Severely myopic disks may have a small degree of temporal pallor. Optic atrophy has seven major features:

1 pallor of the disk; if white (aspirin-like) it denotes disease of the nerve or retinal ganglion cells; if a waxy yellow it is often associated with retinitis pigmentosa;

2 sharp margins;

3 loss of the lamina cribrosa in the cup;

4 increased cup to disk ratio;

5 decreased arterioles off the disk (less than 14);

6 small arteries;

7 gray pale retina.

Some purists demand a decrease of visual acuity with optic atrophy, which is most often the case.

Swelling

Papilledema is characterized by: (Plate 1h, facing page 26)

1 Progressive loss of the disk margin, superior earlier than inferior and lastly temporal. The nasal margins are always slightly blurred.

2 Fat veins with loss of venous pulsations (rarely, venous pulsations can be seen with papilledema).

3 Erythema of the disk.

4 Loss of the lamina cribrosa; the whole cup is pushed forward.

5 Radial streaking or "slit" hemorrhages are noted off the disk margin.

6 Engorged veins appear and disappear near the disk.

7 Folds are noted in the retina which spread toward the macula.

Importantly, visual acuity is normal. The only visual field abnormality is an enlarged blind spot. Chronic papilledema is associated with constricted visual fields.

Papillitis (see Plate 1e, facing page 26) is swelling of the disk from inflammation (multiple sclerosis) or ischemia (giant cell arteritis or hypertension in older patients). Toxins (methanol) or infection (HIV) is suspected (in the presence of associated other signs and symptoms) if the patient has central scotomata with diminution of visual acuity. The veins are not engorged, the disk swelling is less marked and peripapillary hemorrhages and venous sheathing (Rucker's) may be present. The process is often unilateral.

Patients with retrobulbar neuritis present with a central scotomata and periorbital pain exacerbated by ocular movement. The examiner "sees nothing" and the patient sees "nothing."

Foster Kennedy syndrome (Plate 1g, facing page 26) may produce papilledema in one eye and optic atrophy in the other. The usual location of the mass that produces this constellation of signs is the inferior frontal gyrus (olfactory groove) and pathologies include meningioma, glioma and mucocele. The patient has unilateral anosmia (compression of the olfactory nerve) and ipsilateral papilledema with contralateral optic atrophy. The former is caused by obstruction of venous return or increased intracranial pressure and the latter by direct compression of the nerve.

Pseudopapilledema (Plate 1i, facing page 26)

Hypermetropic disks (in an elongated eye) may appear smaller than normal and their margins are blurred. The vessels are normal and venous pulsations are present. Obliquity of the optic nerve head, juxtapapillary choroiditis, drusen bodies, sarcoid and hamartomas of the disk may appear to cause disk swelling. Rarely, abnormal myelination of optic nerve fibers extends into the retina. Venous pulsations and normal vessels distinguish these entities from true papilledema.

Central venous occlusion is usually unilateral and has an abrupt onset. Retinal hemorrhages are central rather than "slit" off the disk, the vessels are engorged and there is loss of vision.

Papilledema occurs in the setting of an increased P_{CO_2} (usually greater than 70 mmHg). This is secondary to dilation of cerebral vessels from H^+ ions (that activate DRASIC receptors which dilate cerebral blood vessels). This phenomenon occurs with neuromuscular diseases with respiratory failure such as myasthenia gravis and Guillain–Barré syndrome (GBS). It may also be seen with severe emphysema or any cause of respiratory failure. Leukemia and severe anemias may be associated with papilledema as a result of leaky cerebral blood vessels.

The vessels

The retina is a window to cerebral and systemic blood vessels. Arteries are smaller than veins and have a light streak. Hypertension, atherosclerosis and diabetes often occur concomitantly and their signature is in the retina. The arteries are thin following ophthalmic artery thrombosis and there is concomitant retinal pallor ("grayness"). Crossing defects, arteries compressing veins, are common with hypertension and atherosclerosis and are often associated with retinal exudates and drusen.

Both arteries and veins are tortuous in the vascular malformation of von Hippel–Lindau disease. This entity is associated with cerebral, cerebellar and spinal malformations as well as renal cell carcinoma, a high hematocrit and excess vascular endothelial growth factor (VEGF).

The retina

The retina and choroid demonstrate multiple abnormalities that are associated with systemic and neurologic disease. Some major neurologic entities that can be identified by evaluation of the retina and choroid are described below.

Hemorrhages (Plate 1f, facing page 26)

Any cause of raised intracranial pressure causes small, flame-shaped or linear streak hemorrhages off the disk as well as larger ecchymoses that obscure blood vessels and the retina. Venous engorgement with hemorrhage occurs from leukemia and high serum immunoglobulin M (IgM). Hypertension and systemic vasculitides cause hemorrhages in the central retina and macula.

Microaneurysms that produce small, round hemorrhages are characteristic of diabetes. Subhyaloid or preretinal hemorrhages occur with subarachnoid bleeding. They are now thought to be caused by the sudden increase of retinal pressure concurrent with the bleed rather than by leakage of blood that seeps under the meninges which cover the optic nerve. They may be seen below or contiguous with the disk, have crescentic inner and clear-cut outer borders that extend toward the lens. They move and change contour with different head positions (Torsten's syndrome).

Exudates

Cotton wool exudates may be seen with papilledema, renal failure, severe hypertension, polyarteritis, systemic lupus erythematosus, severe anemia and embolism. The etiology is a microinfarct of axons with an inflammatory reaction.

Roth spots are embolic infarcts with a clear center and a hemorrhagic surround. Similar findings may be noted with severe hyperthyroidism, anemia or leukemia.

A macular star forms from edema outlining the nerve fiber layer of the macula. It is most often encountered with severe hypertension associated with renal failure. Retinal vasculitis denotes inflammatory changes of or adjacent to retinal vessels. It is denoted by perivascular sheathing of veins and arteries, occlusion and retinal hemorrhages. It is accompanied by cells and protein in the anterior chamber (hypophon) and the vitreous. Some entities have associated uveitis (Behçet's, sarcoid, Vogt–Koyanagi disease). Recently noted are cytomegalovirus infections of the retina in conjunction with HIV. *Bartonella* infection (catscratch disease), syphilis, tuberculosis and Lyme are other infections of retinal blood vessels. Syphilis causes retinitis pigmentosa (RP) adjacent to blood vessels whereas the idiopathic form of RP is scattered throughout the retina. All collagen vascular diseases may be associated with retinal vasculitis as is multiple sclerosis and its variants.

Tubercles

Tubercles may appear on the disk and have been confused with papilledema. In general, they are approximately half of a disk diameter, yellowish in the center with ill-defined pink margins. They are slightly raised and may be associated with RP as is syphilis. In acute miliary tuberculosis, multiple tubercles may be seen in peripheral retinal vessels.

Phakomas

A phakoma is an aggregate of abnormal neurologic cells that are plaque-like

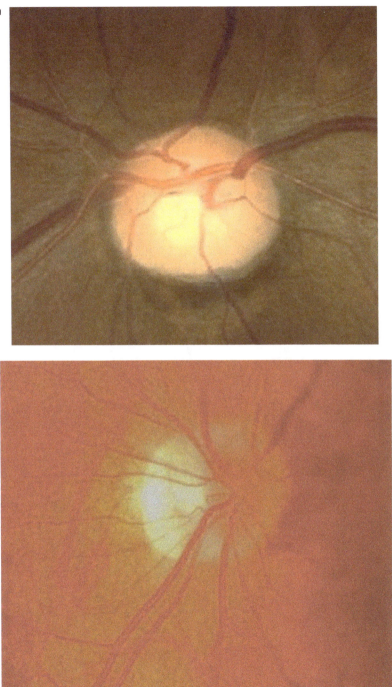

Plate 1 (a) Normal disk. Note the normal color and arteries of the temporal margin. (b) Atrophy of the temporal margin. The macular papillary bundle. The patient had long-standing multiple sclerosis.

1c

1d

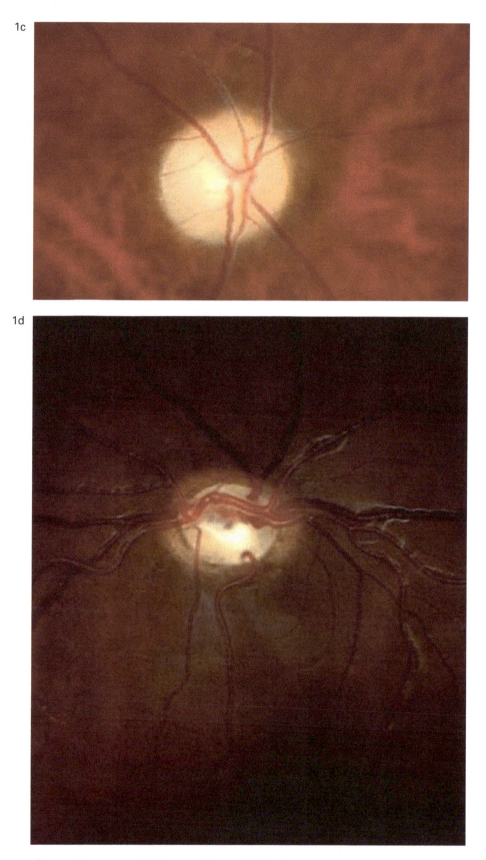

Plate 1 (c) Optic atrophy long-standing multiple sclerosis. (d) Coloboma (congenital defect).

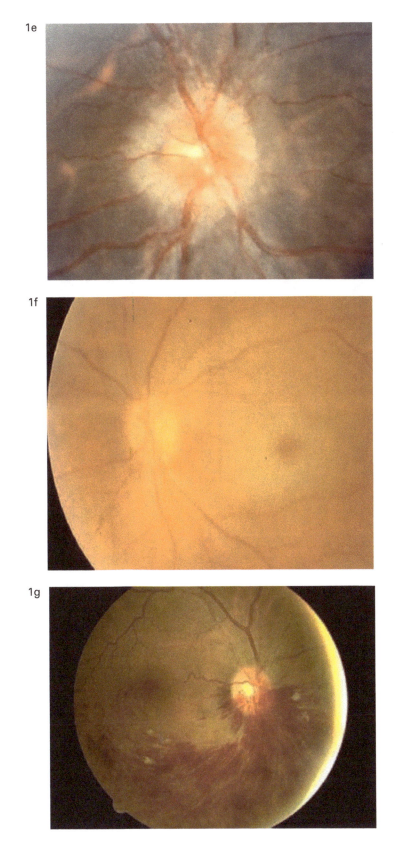

Plate 1 Types of hemorrhages in the disk: (e) Papillitis. (f) Central retinal artery occlusion ischemia. (g) Venous hemorrhage.

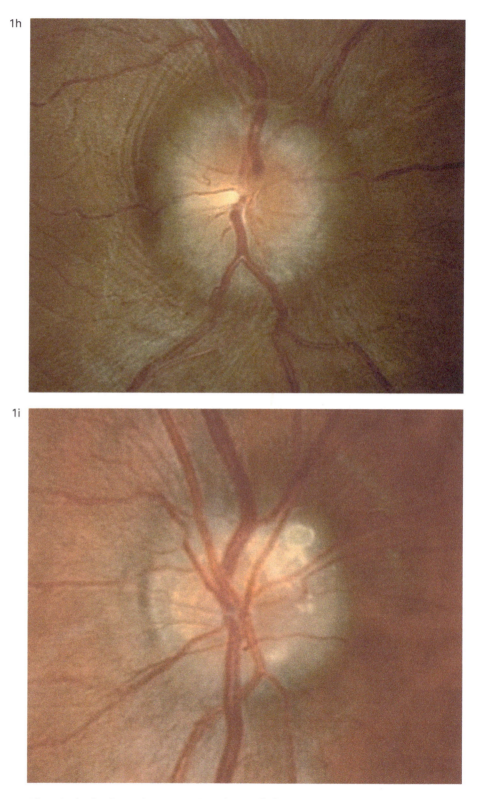

Plate 1 The fundoscopic examination: (h) Papilledema. (i) Pseudopapilledema.

with translucent edges. They are between half and two-thirds of the size of the optic disk. They are usually seen in tuberous sclerosis to a greater degree than neurofibromatosis and may be found in any portion of the retina. Rarely, they occur on the disk and are a cause of pseudopapilledema.

Collagen defects: pigmentary abnormalities

Retinitis pigmentosa is an important pigmentary abnormality to recognize in the retina. It is a spidery black "bone corpuscle" pigmentation that spreads from the periphery to the center of the retina. It is not contiguous with blood vessels as is that associated with neurosyphilis. A similar pattern of migratory pigmentation may be seen in Laurence–Moon–Biedl syndrome (mental retardation, obesity, RP and hyperdactyly), Aicardi's syndrome (seizures, absence of the corpus callosum, two electrically independent hemispheres by EEG), multiple mitochondrial entities including Kearns–Sayre syndrome (ophthalmoplegia, heart block, diabetes mellitus, RP) and many other genetic deficits. In idiopathic RP, the disk is atrophic and waxy yellow as opposed to the aspirin-like disk of primary optic atrophy. In the cerebromacular degenerations, a cherry red spot is caused by degeneration of the retinal ganglion cells that exposes the blood supply of the choroids. The macula is surrounded by granular, peppery-appearing pigment in association with retinal atrophy.

Congenital toxoplasmosis is characterized by large, bilateral, punched out, oval pigmentary abnormalities in and around the macula. In acquired toxoplasmosis, the lesions are usually unilateral.

Myelinated nerve fibers

Myelinated nerve fibers that project into the retina spread from the optic disk, are vividly white, clear-cut and curvilinear. The peripheral edge fades into the retina. These fibers may be mistaken for papilledema or an exudate.

Third, fourth and sixth cranial nerves

Method of examination: inspection

While taking the history, the examiner should evaluate the position of the eyes for esotropia or exotropia, skew deviation, pupillary size, palpebral fissure width, ptosis, exophthalmus and enophthalmos.

Esotropia and exotropia

Comitant esotropia is congenital and the inward deviation of the affected eye is maintained in all fields of gaze. The examiner covers the unaffected eye and straight fixation breaks conjugate gaze which causes the esotropic eye to shift outward the same number of degrees it was off fixation in primary gaze. If the eye does not move outward with the normally fixated eye covered, there is failure of abduction and a sixth nerve palsy.

The same principles apply to an eye that is abducted in primary gaze. If this deviation is comitant it is a congenital defect. If it is non-comitant and the eye is down and slightly out there is a third nerve deficit. Depending where in the course of the third nerve the injury lies will determine if the pupil is involved. In general, medical third nerve palsies spare the pupil. A surgical third nerve palsy is usually caused by a posterior communicating aneurysm which compresses pupillary fibers that are peripheral in the nerve. Another school of thought suggests that pupillary fibers are more pressure sensitive and are affected throughout the nerve. If the eye is pulled in with abduction, there is congenital shortening and fibrosis of the medial rectus muscle or congenital aberrant innervation of the third and sixth nerves (Duane's syndrome).

Vertical squints

The examiner notes that the eyes are not on the same vertical plane. If there is a brainstem lesion, it is on the side of the down eye. If the lesion is above the tentorium, it is often in the opposite thalamus.

If the deviation is upward in primary gaze and the patient cannot look down with the eye in abduction, there is a lesion of the inferior rectus muscle. If the patient cannot look down and in, the problem lies with the fourth cranial nerve. The function of the fourth nerve can only be seen in the presence of a complete third nerve palsy. The eye can be seen to be depressed and inwardly rotated looking down and in.

Exophthalmos

The best way to evaluate exophthalmos is to stand behind the patient and look down. Shallow orbits at times appear to cause ocular protuberance. The examiner should gently assess the tension of the eyes. If there is increased intraorbital pressure, it will be difficult to compress the globe. The exophthalmic eye will be down and in from a lacrimal gland tumor, but straight protuberant with pseudotumor of the orbit (an inflammatory process) and with thyrotoxicosis. This entity is often associated with chemosis (edema) and injection of the conjunctiva. The lids are frequently edematous and there may be oculomotor paresis (thyroid ophthalmopathy). All muscles may be paralyzed, but the lid is normal. Exophthalmos may be severe in craniostenosis but rarely in hydrocephalus.

Unilateral exophthalmos is most often caused by hyperthyroidism. It may also be seen in association with a cavernous carotid fistula where there is conjunctival infection that reaches the iris (arterialized venous blood). In infection, vessels do not extend to the iris. Orbital and retro-orbital neoplasms, hemangiomas, pseudotumor and lacrimal gland tumors all cause unilateral exophthalmos. Unilateral pulsatile exophthalmos is seen in neurofibroma type I resulting from absence of the sphenoid bone. Rarely, a bruit is heard over the eye with a carotid cavernous fistula. Thrombosis and tumors of the cavernous sinus (meningioma, lymphoma, lateral extension of a pituitary adenoma) are associated with third, fourth and sixth nerve palsies as well as exophthalmos. Meningiomas of the medial and lateral sphenoid wing are also associated with unilateral exophthalmos.

Enophthalmos

Enophthalmos may be associated with congenital ocular defects. Minimally apparent enophthalmos is most common with Horner's syndrome. There is sympathetically innervated smooth muscle in the tarsal plates of the lid and a few slips of smooth muscle posterior to the globe (Müller's muscle). Careful observation reveals not only ptosis with Horner's syndrome, but a subtle elevation of the lower lid. Scirrhous carcinoma from the breast metastatic to the orbit causes significant enophthalmos. Enophthalmos with abduction of the eye suggests congential fibrosis of the medial rectus muscle or aberrant connections between the third and sixth nerve.

Hypertelorism

Many normal individuals have hypertelorism. In neurologic practice it should alert the examiner to a congenital absence of the corpus callosum, Aicardi's syndrome or Schapiro's syndrome (hypothermia and other hypo-thalamic defects as well as a host of congenital defects). Less frequently noted is hypotelorism, which is most often seen in septo-optic dysplasia. In this condition, there is optic nerve hypoplasia and a small sella turcica with pituitary dysfunction.

The conjunctiva

Subconjunctival hemorrhages are common with head trauma and rare in subarachnoid hemorrhage and severe hypertension. Leptospirosis (*Leptospira canicola*) causes an inflammatory conjunctival reaction with injection of blood vessels in association with meningitis and myopathy. Conjunctival injection is prominent during the migratory phase of filaria (*Loa loa*), which may also be associated with meningitis.

Telangiectasia of the conjunctiva may be a feature of sickle cell (SS) disease. They are also characteristic of ataxia telangiectasia and are associated with cutaneous lesions of the flexor creases of the forearm. They may be noted at 1 year of age. Ataxia, basal ganglia dysfunction, mental retardation and lymphoma are seen in conjunction with ataxia in this entity.

Retro-orbital tumors may grow forwards and produce a red or gray subconjunctival discoloration noted on extreme deviation of the globe.

Renal failure is associated with severe conjunctival injection. Tears are alkaline and the general acidosis of renal failure causes an intense inflammatory conjunctival reaction. The conjunctiva may be faintly yellow in systemic or metastatic liver failure.

The cornea and iris

Shy–Drager syndrome is associated with an atrophic iris. The iris of a patient with congenital Horner's syndrome is blue while its mate may be brown. The tabetic iris is pale and atrophied. Aniridia may be seen as a component of a form of hereditary sensory autonomic neuropathy. Iris atrophy appears to cause a deep anterior chamber which is fenestrated.

The Kayser–Fleischer ring (Wilson's disease) is one of a very few pathognomonic signs in medicine. Most often it is a golden-brown ring inside the limbus of the cornea that may form a complete circle or just a crescent at the upper and lower margins. It is difficult to see in dark eyes. Slitlamp evaluation reveals copper deposition in Desçemet's membrane. After treatment with penicillamine it becomes a dull mottled brown. Behçet's, Kawasaki's and Stevens–Johnson syndrome can all produce conjunctival ulcers as do all severe collagen vascular diseases.

The eyelids

The position of the lids in relation to the iris and the width of the palpebral fissure are noted in primary gaze and with forced eye opening. The lid movement and concomitant degree of frontalis muscle action are noted. The patient is then asked to follow an object upwards and hold gaze for 30–45 seconds without blinking.

Ptosis

If the upper lid covers the top of the iris, there may be weakness of the levator palpebrae superioris muscle from a third nerve lesion or weakness of the sympathetically innervated tarsal muscles within the upper lid. If this is the case, the patient can voluntarily raise the lid. If the third nerve is involved, the frontalis muscle contracts to compensate. The lower lid also elevates with sympathetic denervation of its tarsal muscle. This is a very helpful sign in older patients with droopy eyelids.

In myasthenia gravis the lid droop varies and increases with prolonged up gaze. A blink restores it to its normal position. A slight ptosis may be noted in the contralateral eye. The pupils are normal to clinical examination.

In the ocular myopathies (dystrophic, congenital and mitochondrial) the ptosis is fixed and the head is often extended to look out under the drooping lids. The ptosis tends to be symmetric in these entities.

Lid retraction

Pathologic lid retraction (Collier's sign) occurs in a variety of central and peripheral conditions. The lid should follow the globe in up and down gaze in a yoked fashion. If the sclerae is seen above the iris on down gaze, there is pathologic lid retraction. This occurs on a peripheral basis most commonly with hyperthyroidism, but may also be noted with excess anticholinesterase medication, hypokalemic periodic paralysis and in any state that results in a high concentration of circulating norepinephrine such as metastatic liver disease (norepinephrine cannot be metabolized).

On a central basis, the central caudal nucleus of the third nerve complex innervates the levator palpebrae superioris which is at the level of the red nucleus and may be irritated from a mass lesion which causes pathologic lid retraction on down gaze or Collier's sign.

The pupils

Pupils need to be evaluated for size, shape, equality and regularity. Pupillary size in normal ambient light in a fully awake patient varies from 2 to 4 mm. If the patient has ingested amphetamines, cocaine or there is excessive circulating norepinephrine, often from anoxia, they may dilate to 5–6 mm. A lesion at the thalamic basal ganglion level produces a 2–3 mm pupil that is responsive to light and accommodation. There are two major pupil sizes at midbrain levels. A cadaveric pupil is 3 mm and is not responsive to light or accommodation. A pretectal pupil is 3–4 mm and is minimally reactive to light, but is compatible with life. A severely compromised midbrain may cause maximally dilated 6 mm pupils. An elliptical pupil ("cat's eye pupil") is often seen after midbrain damage from head trauma. An oval pupil may be seen with third nerve damage anywhere in its course. It is also seen in partial peripheral third nerve damage from compression or infarction. Pontine pupils from any pathology, usually hemorrhage that destroys sympathetic afferent innervation, are 0.5 mm in diameter but constrict to light. A Horner's pupil is usually 1 mm and light reactive. Pupils are small in early infancy, old age, during sleep and in bright light. They are large in poor illumination, myopia and childhood.

Reaction to light

The patient is instructed to fix on a distant object (to block accommodation), preferably in a dim room. A bright light is applied from the side, which should initiate a brisk pupillary constriction. The two sides are compared and should be equal in size and reactivity. The consensual response is elicited by shining the light in one eye which elicits constriction in the contralateral eye. This reflex is integrated in the midbrain pretectal area.

Reaction to convergence and accommodation for near vision

The patient fixes on a distant object and then is asked to look at an object 22 cm in front of the bridge of the nose. The patient is asked to refixate on the distant object, which causes pupillary dilation, which may be easier to evaluate.

Pupillary abnormalities

The constricted pupil (miosis)

The small pupil is usually caused by interruption of the sympathetic innervation of the pupillary dilator muscle. The frontal eye fields in area 6 are a major source of bilateral cortical projections to the sympathetic system. Lesions here may cause either ipsilateral or contralateral ptosis and meiosis (so-called "baby Horner's"). These cortical fibers project to the posterior hypothalamus where a decussation occurs. The sympathetic fibers travel laterally in the thalamus, midbrain and medulla (and are often affected in Wallenberg's lateral medullary infarction) to synapse as far down as the T2 thoracic level. The major sympathetic supply to the eye is from the C8–T1 spinal segments (ciliary center of Budge). The sympathetic innervation of the arm is primarily from T2. After synapsing in the cervical and thoracic spinal segments, sympathetic afferents synapse in the superior cervical sympathetic ganglia, wrap around the carotid artery in the pericarotid plexus and reach the eye by accompanying the ophthalmic division of the fifth nerve.

Horner's syndrome can occur from a lesion anywhere in the pathway. In general, lesions proximal to the superior cervical ganglia (i.e., brainstem or intraparenchymal lesions) are much less evident than peripheral lesions. Central lesions do not cause as much pupillary dilation to mydriatics as those distal to the superior cervical ganglia (Cannon's law; i.e., there will be up-regulation of adrenoreceptors from the distal denervating lesion). A lesion anywhere in this pathway will cause miosis. Pontine lesions, carotid surgery, sulcal lung tumors, hypothalamic strokes or any lesion of the sympathetic chain causes miosis. Primary autonomic failure, multiple system atrophy and some familial causes also demonstrate miotic pupils. Bilateral sympathetic lesions are most often seen with upper brainstem lesions. A sleeping patient, even if the eyes are not completely closed, may have very small pupils which dilate rapidly with arousal.

Horner's syndrome

The complete syndrome consists of:
1 miosis;
2 ptosis;
3 apparent enophthalmos;
4 anidrosis and warmth of the face.
Cocaine will not dilate the pupil (mechanism of its action is blockade of reuptake of dopamine and noradrenaline) and adrenaline dilates it more than usual (Cannon's law of denervation supersensitivity). A lesion of the

common carotid artery alone will spare the sympathetic supply to the face (travels with the external carotid artery) and a lesion of the carotid bifurcation will cause a complete Horner's as both the eye and facial sympathetic innervation are lesioned. The most obvious peripheral Horner's occurs from lesions of the superior cervical ganglia and carotid artery. A particularly important cause is squamous cell carcinoma of the lung which destroys the sympathetic chain in the thorax. It is rarely noted following carotid catheterization, but is common with severe migraine (Raeder's paratrigeminal neuralgia), cluster headache and the autonomic trigeminal migraine syndromes. It is a cardinal sign of carotid dissection in association with contralateral hemiparesis and facial pain.

The central Horner's syndromes are noted most commonly with Wallenberg's syndrome, but may be seen with any lateral brainstem lesion.

A "baby Horner's" may occur following lesions of the frontal eye fields. This is usually noted as ptosis (decreased cortical innervation to the central caudal nucleus of the third nerve complex) most often ipsilaterally, but at times contralaterally with minimal miosis (decreased cortical–diencephalic innervation) which also occurs ipsi- and contralaterally.

Dilated pupil (mydriasis)

A dilated pupil is caused by lesions of the parasympathetic nuclei and fibers in the midbrain third nerve complex (rare), in association with the third nerve and cerebral peduncle (Weber's syndrome), dentatorubral thalamic system (Benedict's and Claude's syndromes), compression by the uncus of the hippocampal gyrus (herniation) or compression under the posterior communicating artery with hemispheric swelling. The third nerve with pupillary involvement occurs in cavernous sinus lesions in association with involvement of the fourth, fifth and sixth nerve. The pupil tends to be more involved with anterior cavernous sinus lesions. In the orbit, the pupillary fibers course with the inferior division of the third nerve which also innervates the inferior rectus muscle. There have been debates as to the exact location of the parasympathetic pupillary constrictor fibers. Some authorities believe that they are superficial within the third nerve between 12 and 3 o'clock, while others suggest that these fibers are scattered equally throughout the nerve, but are pressure sensitive.

In general, medical causes of third nerve palsy cause severe ptosis, but spare the pupil. Surgical causes of compression of the third nerve such as a posterior communicating or carotid aneurysm affect the pupil and cause less severe ptosis. An eye that is almost amaurotic may have a dilated pupil as does one that has recently been dilated with a mydriatic.

The pupil that does not react to light

The lesion in this instance may be in the retina (ganglion cell loss), optic nerve or chiasm or the parasympathetic nerve supply that courses with the third nerve. In anterior lesions, there will be no consensual reaction in the unaffected eye as no light can trigger the midbrain pretectal reflex. If the lesion is unilateral (optic neuritis or partial compression), light shone into the normal eye causes both pupils to contract. In bilateral lesions there is no consensual response if either side is stimulated. Bilateral failure of the consensual light reflex with normal visual acuity localizes the lesion to the midbrain.

The "swinging flash light" test is important in patients with demyelinating disease. A bright light is shone into the normal eye, which causes bilateral pupillary constriction. It is then switched to the affected eye, which dilates in the face of direct light. This is known as an afferent pupillary defect (APD) and many feel it is caused by damage of the optic nerve. Others have pointed out the great sensitivity of the reflex, which may be triggered by a few myelinated fibers, which certainly survive an attack of optic neuritis. The afferent pupillary defect is thus thought to be "slippage" of the midbrain consensual reflex. The mechanism notwithstanding, it is a reliable test to determine a defect in one optic nerve. Color desaturation and lack of phosphenes (colored lights) after a bright light are confirmatory. Bilateral blindness with non-reacting pupils is brought about by a lesion between the retina and the first part of the optic tract, because after this point pupilloconstrictor fibers have diverged from visual fibers.

The pupil that fails to accommodate for near vision and light near dissociation

This phenomenon is almost always caused by pressure or destruction of the midbrain as a result of a tumor. More commonly, light near dissociation is seen. This is a pupil that responds to accommodation to a greater degree than it does to light. This may be seen in autonomic failures (such as multiple system atrophy), diabetic autonomic neuropathy and amyloid neuropathy. It is an excellent reflex to evaluate in an elderly patient with hypotension or mild cognitive impairment (multiple system atrophy).

Argyll Robertson pupil

Since the advent of HIV and consequent syphilitic infections, this pupillary defect has made a strong comeback. It has five major components:
1 small;
2 irregular;
3 responds to accommodation;
4 does not respond to light;
5 does not respond to mydriatics.

It is occasionally seen in midbrain lesions (tectum). Some favor the ciliary ganglion as the site of the lesion. The pupils are not always small and may not be symmetrical.

Myotonic pupil (Holmes–Adie syndrome)

This is a syndrome that is primarily seen in young women. It is usually discovered when the young lady is applying cosmetics. One pupil is noted to be larger than the other. On examination, it fails to react to light but does to accommodation. There is concomitant loss of ankle and knee jerks. Occasionally, patients are areflexic. Formerly the lesion was thought to occur in the ciliary ganglion, but now the condition is felt to be a generalized neuropathy. The most characteristic feature of the syndrome is the slow constriction of the pupil with maintained convergence. The dilation of the pupil is slow when the patient fixes gaze on a distant object. A small dose of parasympathomimetics (2.5%) will cause a brisk response, demonstrating denervation supersensitivity.

Behr's pupil

Behr's is a slightly dilated pupil in association with an optic tract lesion that is usually associated with a contralateral hemiparesis. A glioma is the usual pathology.

Wernicke's pupil

This is the purview of the neurophthalmologist. The pathology is usually a stroke that damages the optic tract, leaving the patient with a non-congruent hemianopsia. A slit lamp directed to the sighted field elicits a pupillary response which does not occur in the blind component of the field.

Examining ocular movement (Fig. 3.5)

This part of the neurologic examination defeats a great number of examiners. It is easy if the following rules are observed:
1 Note the deviation of the eyes in primary gaze. If an eye muscle is weak, its yoked partner will pull the eye in its direction of action.
2 Place the eye in a position such that the affected muscle can be tested in its primary field of action. Almost everything happens to the third and sixth nerve.
3 A fourth nerve deficit is almost always accompanied by a head deviation to the contralateral side.

The patient is asked to follow the finger which is moved right and left horizontally, upwards and downwards in the midline. Each deviation should be held for a few seconds. The examiner notes lagging of one or the other eye, diplopia and nystagmus.

The analysis of eye movements, nystagmus conjugate gaze is extremely helpful in topical diagnosis and is very easy.

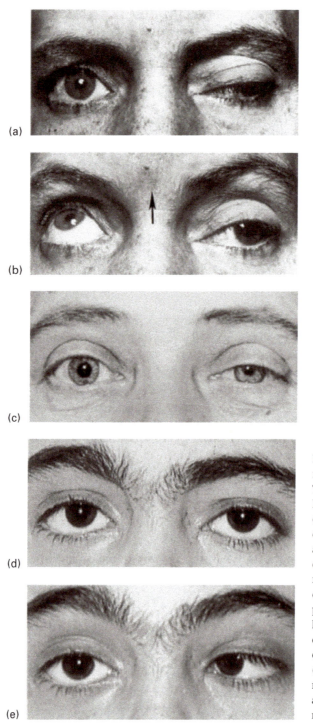

(a)

(b)

(c)

(d)

(e)

Fig. 3.5 Extraocular movements. (a) Partial left Third nerve palsy. Ptosis and lateral deviation of the left eye. (b) Upward gaze; slight elevation of the left lid reveals a dilated pupil and paralysis of elevation of the left eyeball; note hypermetria of the right eye. (c) Horner's syndrome; ptosis, elevation of the lower lid, miosis, slight enophthalmos; no overaction of the frontis muscle. (d) and (e) Sixth nerve paralysis. The right eye is deviated inwards and cannot abduct to cross the midline.

Actions of the ocular muscles

A   The external rectus (sixth nerve), moves the eye horizontally outwards (abduction). If weak, the eye is adducted in primary gaze.

B   The internal rectus (third nerve), moves the eye horizontally inwards (adduction).

C   The superior rectus (third nerve), elevates the eye when it is abducted.

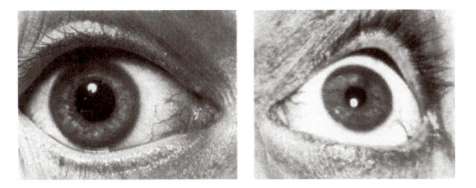

Fig. 3.6 Kayser–Fleischer ring.

D The inferior oblique (third nerve), elevates the eye when it is adducted.

E The inferior rectus (third nerve), depresses the eye when it is abducted.

F The superior oblique (fourth nerve), depresses and internally rotates the eye when it is adducted. The internal rotation can only be seen if there is a concomitant complete third nerve palsy.

If the eye is in (esotropia) on primary gaze the examiner suspects a sixth nerve palsy. The face is slightly turned to the side of the sixth nerve deficit. Rarely, there may be a deficit of the external rectus muscle (fibrosis).

If the adducted eye cannot move downwards, is hyperopic in primary gaze, there is a fourth nerve lesion or a local lesion of the superior oblique muscle. There is a contralateral head tilt. The head is performing the depressor function usually accomplished by the superior oblique muscle and fourth nerve.

All other deficits of ocular movements are caused by third nerve lesions. These include a local pathology of muscles, myasthenia gravis and mitochondrial, dystrophic or genetic myopathies, an internuclear ophthalmoplegia (Fig. 3.6) or conjugate gaze center lesion. All of the above have clear identifying features.

Incomplete paralysis of ocular muscle may be difficult to see by examination so the patient's diplopia will then need to be evaluated.

Analysis of diplopia

A few simple rules need to be remembered.

1 The angle of incidence equals the angle of reflectance. If the eye is deviated as a result of muscle weakness, the light ray will be reflected from a direct course to the fovea by the lens to the same degree as the deviation that was caused by the weak muscle. Thus, a sixth nerve lesion would cause the eye in primary gaze to be deviated inwards in adduction by the intact medial rectus. The light ray would be reflected laterally to the fovea and the false image would be lateral to the image that was perceived from the normal eye. The fovea has the greatest concentration of cones, which record color, and determines resolution. The light reflected off the lens falls on retina that subserves rod vision (primarily for motion and not resolution). The false image is paler and less distinct.

2   Separation of the images is greatest in the field of gaze in which the weak muscle has it purest action.

3   The false image is displaced furthest in the direction in which the weak muscle moves the eye (laterally for the medial and lateral recti, vertically for the superior, inferior recti and the superior oblique).

Method of examination

One eye is covered with a red piece of plastic so that any image from this eye is red.

1   In each field of gaze the patient is asked if he or she sees one object or two. At the time it is helpful for the patient to represent what he or she sees with the fingers (i.e., to mimic the images) as they are displaced with movement. The patient is asked if the images are horizontal or vertically displaced.

2   In which position is the image furthest apart?

3   Which one is the red image?

4   Cover one eye and ask the patient to tell which image disappeared.

Interpretation of results

If the images are side by side the medial or lateral recti are defective. If there is a vertical displacement of the images either oblique or the superior and inferior recti are involved.

Muscle pair involved

The position in which there is maximum displacement of the images determines the pair of muscles that are involved. Horizontal displacement on right lateral gaze (right eye covered by red plastic) the red image is most lateral (if the lateral rectus is involved). If the eyes are deviated to the right and upwards, the right superior rectus (red image) and the left inferior oblique are yoked and the separated image will be red (if the superior rectus is weak).

Individual muscle responsible

The image that is furthest displaced from a yoked pair is coming from the weak muscle. This is identified by the color of the image. The false image is always displaced the furthest and is less distinct.

In neurologic practice, most of the time it will be a muscle innervated by the third nerve. Only trauma, diabetes, rarely a metastasis or surgical procedure around the tentorium injures the fourth nerve. Failure to completely abduct the globe (some sclera showing laterally) identifies the sixth nerve as causative of lateral muscle weakness.

Diplopia at near gaze is a third nerve palsy, downward gaze a fourth palsy and far gaze a sixth nerve palsy. This is an excellent rule, but unfortunately it rarely helps in practice.

Common causes of oculomotor paralysis

Third nerve lesions are generally divided into medical or surgical causes. The pupillary involvement and the degree of ptosis are helpful in differentiating the two. Medical third nerve lesions spare the pupil (not strictly true if the examiner uses a magnifying lens) and have a greater degree of ptosis (infarction of the nerve). Bilateral symmetrical ptosis and pupillary paralysis, inability to look up in abduction constitutes a nuclear third nerve (a rare vascular lesion). Symmetrical ptosis and oculomotor weakness is characteristic of mitochondrial disease (Kearns–Sayre syndrome, progressive external ophthalmoplegia), congenital myopathy (centronuclear or myotubular myopathy) and oculopharyngeal dystrophy.

Isolated third nerve lesions may occur with branch occlusion of the posterior cerebral artery. Most often these occur with contralateral weakness (fascicular third nerve) or with ataxia (Claude's syndrome) or choreoathetosis (Benedict's syndrome) from thalamoperforate branch occlusion of the P1 segment of the posterior cerebral artery. Rarely, a rather isolated third nerve can be seen with an ascending interpeduncular branch occlusion from the top of the basilar artery. Myasthenia gravis frequently affects the third nerve with pupillary sparing and increased ptosis with fatigue. Rarely, demyelinating disease affects the third nerve.

A surgical third nerve is seen with posterior communicating, carotid and superior cerebellar aneurysms, large aneurysms at the top of the basilar (often in conjunction with the fourth nerve), parasellar neoplasms, medial sphenoid wing meningiomas and skull-based tumors.

The sixth nerve has a long intracranial course and is involved in many conditions that affect the base of the skull. These include all forms of meningitis, metastatic lesions and skull-based tumors. Intraparenchymal involvement occurs with pontine strokes (often in conjunction with a nuclear seventh nerve palsy), the Millard–Gubler syndrome. In isolation or with a contralateral hemiparesis it is Ramon's syndrome. It may be trapped unilaterally or bilaterally under the petroclinoid ligament (Dorello's canal at the petrous apex) with acute increased intracranial pressure (a false localizing sign).

Fourth nerve lesions are very rare and are most commonly seen with head trauma and diabetes.

Paralysis of the third, fourth, sixth and nerve V_1 comprise the cavernous sinus syndrome. This is most often brought about by meningioma, lymphoma or aneurysm of the carotid artery or thrombosis of the sinus.

Conjugate ocular movement (Figs 3.7 and 3.8)

The new methods of "clot busting" with both intravenous and intra-arterial

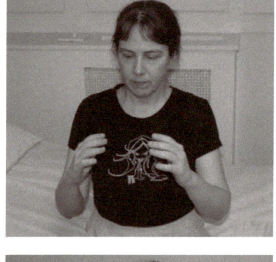

(a)

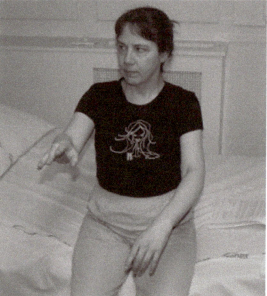

(b)

Fig. 3.7 (a) Normally, the left frontal fields conjugately deviate the eyes to the right and vice versa. (b) Right-sided lesions of the frontal eye fields with left hemiparesis.

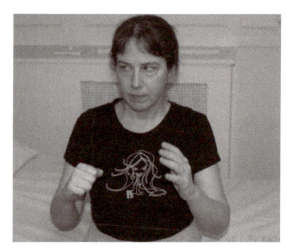

Fig. 3.8 Right parapontine reticular formation center lesion. The eyes are pulled to the left. The hemiparesis is on the left.

tissue plasminogen activator (tPA) or urokinase, angioplasty and stenting have dramatically changed stroke therapy. This aspect of neurology is now treatable and it is incumbent upon all to understand this concept and to act immediately. There is presently a time window of 3 hours for intravenous therapy and 6 hours for intra-arterial tPA therapy. Conjugate eye deviation helps the emergency room physician, internist and neurologist to quickly assess the artery involved, the pathology of the stroke and the correct treatment.

The cortical center for conjugate gaze is located in area 6 of the frontal lobe (frontal eye fields). The right cortical center, if stimulated, initiates conjugate deviation to the left. The neuroanatomic basis of horizontal eye movement is as follows. Area 7 neurons of the parietal lobe ("area of interest" cells) activate the right frontal eye fields. The parapontine reticular formation (PPRF) located ventral to the sixth nerve in the lower third of the pons effects horizontal gaze. Cortical efferents from the right frontal eye fields project to the globus pallidus (GPI) and superior colliculus which in turn activate burst neurons of the left PPRF, which move the eyes horizontally to the left. "Sustaining" neurons of the PPRF keep the eyes (foveated) on the target. To move conjugately to the right, the right sixth nerve must contract (the left is inhibited) and the left medial rectus must contract (the right is inhibited). There are cortical fixation reflexes that project to "sustaining" neurons of the PPRF that also help maintain fixation. These pathways are also activated reflexly from the vestibular nuclei (superior, inferior and medial) that project to the occipital and frontal eye fields. The third and sixth nerves are linked (yoked) by the medial longitudinal fasciculus (MLF). There is heavy innervation from the vestibular nuclei of the brainstem to the MLF. There are also heavy projections from the proprioceptive fibers of cervical vertebrae to the vestibular nuclei (spinovestibular tract).

The system is modulated and eye movements are smoothed out by the cerebellum. The system appears to be complicated, but it is not (see Figs 3.7 and 3.8). If there is a lesion of the left frontal eye fields (FEF), the right FEF will dominate and the eyes will be deviated to the left. The hemiparesis (arm and face greater than leg) will be on the right (the FEF is subserved by an arterial supply that overlaps with that of the motor strip for the arm and face). To avoid confusion, the examiner should hold his or her hands in front with the index fingers opposed. Thus, if the right side is damaged, the left wins and the eyes are conjugately deviated to the right.

The PPRF of the lower third of the pons is organized differently. Each side pulls the eye to the ipsilateral side. If the right side is damaged, the eyes will be deviated to the left forever and will not be able to cross the midline with any form of stimulation. The hemiparesis will be on the side of the lesion. To avoid confusion, the examiner places his or her fist in front with the thumb abducted also. The corticospinal tract decussates at C1–C2 on the same side; thus, the hemiparesis is on the same side as the eye deviation. The eyes and hemiparesis are on the side of the lesion with brainstem strokes that affect the center for horizontal gaze.

The conjugate center for up gaze is in the midbrain at the level of the superior colliculus in the midbrain ocular area. It is the rostral interstitial nucleus of the MLF (riMLF). Its ventral neurons subserve down gaze. In general, structural lesions that compress the midbrain cause downward deviation of the eyes usually only 5–10°. If the patient appears to be looking at the tip of their nose, this is most often a thalamic lesion which compresses the center for up gaze or disrupts these fibers before they reach the midbrain. One eye down and in also suggests a thalamic lesion on the side opposite the eye.

The area of interest cells of the parietal posterior cortex (area 7) project to the frontal eye fields which then initiate vertical gaze by projections to the riMLF and superior colliculus. The oblique and recti muscles are coordinated to affect downward or upward gaze by the MLF as they are for horizontal gaze. In an unconscious patient, downward conjugate deviation of the eyes suggests a structural rather than a metabolic lesion (pressure on the midbrain center for up gaze).

The centers for smooth pursuit of an object of interest are thought to be occipital. One occipital lobe can effect smooth pursuit of a moving object. The occipital lobe is important for ocular fixation reflexes and has major input from the vestibular nuclei and the floccular nodular lobe of the cerebellum. Unconscious patients with "roving eye movements" have lost their fixation reflexes. "Too easily obtainable" (doll's eye movements) are also a manifestation of loss of cortical fixation reflexes.

Rarely, irritative lesions of the frontal eye fields (seizures) deviate the eyes to the opposite side. Fast components of jerk nystagmus are noted to the side opposite the seizure. Irritative lesions of the brainstem (encephalitis, anoxia, vascular) may drive the eyes to the side of the lesion.

Failure of up gaze in an awake patient is most often caused by a pineal region tumor, vascular accident (branch of the posterior cerebral artery), third ventricular tumor or incipient herniation. Upward herniation of the cerebellar vermis from posterior fossa mass lesions compresses the tectal plate and the riMLF (the eyes will be conjugately deviated downwards). Fixed upward deviation in an awake patient suggests oculogyric crisis from drugs (usually a phenothiazine derivative).

An awake patient who can cooperate but who demonstrates failure of conjugate eye movement in any direction, is instructed to fix his or her eyes on a distant object while the examiner turns the head side to side (to evaluate horizontal gaze) and flexes and extends it (to evaluate vertical gaze). If the ocular deviation is from a metabolic or congenital lesion, the eyes will deviate throughout their full range (vestibular ocular reflex is intact) although the patient cannot do so voluntarily. If a lesion is at the level of the PPRF or the riMLF, the eyes will fail to cross the midline (PPRF) in the former or move vertically (riMLF) in the latter. FEF deviations can be overcome usually within 12 hours by using vestibular ocular reflexes. This is very helpful in deciding the location of ocular deviation in an acute patient.

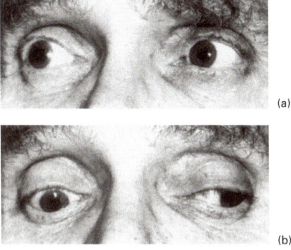

Fig. 3.9 Internuclear ophthalmoplegia. (a) Ocular deviation to the right is normal. (b) To the left, internal deviation of the right eye is defective and the eye turns downwards, external deviation of the left eye is dissociated and accompanied by marked nystagmus.

(a)

(b)

Internuclear ophthalmoplegia

The third and sixth nerve nuclei are connected by the medial longitudinal fasciculus. The decussation is posterior close to the PPRF. Fibers that mediate accommodation are anterior (and innervate the third nerve).

A complete internuclear ophthalmoplegia is illustrated (Fig. 3.9) to right lateral gaze. The components are:

1 nystagmus of the abducting eye;
2 failure to cross the midline (or lag) of the adducting eye;
3 upbeat nystagmus;
4 failure to converge if the lesion is anterior (third nerve area).

If the failure of adduction is complete, the problem is usually an infarction of a penetrating branch of the basilar artery. Less complete lesions are usually caused by demyelinating disease or a vasculitic process. If convergence is maintained, the lesion is posterior at the decussation of the MLF (one of Cogan's laws). The pupils are not involved.

A bilateral internuclear ophthalmoparesis is most often brought about by multiple sclerosis, rarely by systemic lupus erythematosus. Pseudo-internuclear ophthalmoparesis occurs with myasthenia gravis, muscle disease and pressure on the pons.

Detecting and analyzing nystagmus

The eyes at rest are in the midline because of a balance of tone that is maintained from the retina, eye muscles, vestibular nuclei and proprioceptive input from cervical joints and muscles. Unequal input causes a drift of the eyes in a specific direction that is corrected by a quick movement back to the original position. The slow vestibular component of the drift is not seen, but the corrective quick movement is noted and determines the naming of the nystagmus. If this cycle of drift and correction is repeated, it is nystagmus. The various forms of nystagmus are very easy to identify and are extremely helpful in the localization of deficits in the brainstem.

Methods of testing

Nystagmus of primary gaze is frequently noted during history taking. It may be constant or occur in bursts. Instruct the patient to follow the index finger in all fields of gaze. Lateral deviation should be maintained for at least 3 seconds to allow nystagmus to develop. Extreme lateral gaze may break fusion (adducting eye cannot see over the nose) and cause a spurious nystagmus. The lateral or upward movements should not be at the extremes of the field of gaze to avoid this problem.

The examiner notes the following:

1   the position of the eyes that elicits nystagmus;
2   the movement that produces its greatest amplitude, usually to the side of the quick component;
3   the direction of the fast component.

Presenting types of nystagmus

Pendular nystagmus is a rapid horizontal oscillation to either side of the midline with equal amplitude, variable speed that is present on primary gaze. It is increased by fixation, but may lose its pendular quality on lateral gaze. The causes are macular defects, albinism, chorioretinitis, high infantile myopia and opacities of the vitreous.

Congenital nystagmus is pendular in primary, up and down gaze. It has a null point at approximately 14° to the left or right of fixation. Patients have their heads turned to this degree, which helps maintain the image on the fovea. It increases its frequency on lateral gaze.

Horizontal nystagmus ("jerk nystagmus")

The vestibular phase of nystagmus is a slow drift to the side of the lesion. The quick component is a cortical correction. Thus, horizontal jerk nystagmus to the left from a brainstem lesion implies less vestibular input from the right (medical inferior and superior nuclei or their connections) to the third and sixth nuclei such that the left-sided vestibular input drives the eyes to the right (slow phase) but the right frontal conjugate eye center corrects with a quick movement to the left to bring the eyes to mid position.

"Jerk nystagmus" is produced by an imbalance anywhere in the vestibular system or its connections. Thus, it may occur peripherally (i.e., solely from labyrinthine or cervical joints, muscle afferents or eighth nerve input to the vestibular nuclei, or centrally). Common causes of central lesions are at the nuclei, their connections, the medial longitudinal fasciculus, the PPRF (often from drugs that interfere with sustaining neurons which hold fixation on the fovea) and lesions of the cerebellum (involvement of cerebello-vestibular connections). High cervical segment lesions (C1–C4) represent cervicogenic nystagmus (an imbalance of proprioceptive input to vestibular nuclei).

Peripheral lesions are characterized by the fast component beating away from the lesion with the greater amplitude in the direction of the quick phase. Peripheral lesions are usually accompanied by vertigo, tinnitus, nausea and vomiting. Involvement of the eighth nerve from tumor or of the cochlear mechanism from Ménière's disease may be associated with deafness.

In cerebellar lesions or its brainstem connections, the quick phase with greater amplitude is to the side of the lesion. In cerebellar pontine angle tumors, a rotary component with a quick phase is seen to the side of the lesion with a lower amplitude horizontal jerk nystagmus to the side opposite the lesion (pressure from brainstem torque on the opposite center for horizontal gaze (PPRF) in the pons), therefore the eyes are pulled away from this side with the corrective fast phase to the opposite normal side.

In general, central lesions (stroke, multiple sclerosis or low-grade tumors) cause less tinnitus, deafness, vertigo, nausea and vomiting. They also are accompanied by other cranial nerve or long tract deficits.

Vertical nystagmus

Upbeat nystagmus is caused by lesions of the pontomedullary junction or the superior vermis. Downbeat nystagmus accentuated on lateral gaze is secondary to posterior fossa lesions or degenerative diseases such as multiple system atrophy (olivoponto-cerebellar atrophy). Vertical nystagmus from structural lesions, up- and downbeat, is overwhelmingly caused by brainstem disease such as multiple sclerosis, syringobulbia (syrinx is usually lateral under the vestibular nuclei), vertebral artery disease, encephalitis, basilar invagination (odontoid process compression of the medulla) or tonsillar herniation with Chiari malformations. Drugs are the most common cause of vertical (and horizontal) nystagmus by interfering with sustaining neurons of the riMLF and PPRF. The most common are barbiturates, anticonvulsants and benzodiazepines.

Rotary nystagmus

Rotary nystagmus occurs in both labyrinthine, brainstem and eighth nerve disease. The examiner fixes on a small blood vessel of the conjunctiva, which makes the rotary component of the nystagmus easier to see. It is an acute phenomenon with peripheral disorders and is transient. If seen chronically, it implies a lesion of the vestibular nuclei (often the inferior nucleus). All disorders that cause vertical nystagmus can cause rotary nystagmus.

Rare forms of nystagmus

See-saw nystagmus. This is spontaneous movement upwards of one eye with excyclotropia (rotation is counterclockwise) while the contralateral eye moves downward with incyclotropia. This type of nystagmus is seen with parasellar and anterior third ventricle lesions.

Nystagmus retractorius. The eyes move inwards and outwards. The examiner notes subtle widening and narrowing of the palpebral fissures. It is best observed standing to the side of the patient. It is seen with periaqueductal lesions (cysts, gliomas and hemorrhage). It occurs from spontaneous contraction of all extraocular muscles simultaneously.

Convergent-retraction nystagmus. Attempted up gaze, often incomplete, initiates jerk nystagmus with an inward fast convergent phase. This form of nystagmus may be caused by intraventricular (third ventricle) shunts, pineal and midbrain tumors.

Optokinetic nystagmus. This is a normal phenomenon that stabilizes images of stationary objects on the retina during head movement. Either normal occipital lobe can smoothly track a moving target. Once the target is tracked out of the field of gaze (objects moving from left to right), a new object appearing in the left field has to be tracked. This is accomplished by the FEF, which generates a left saccade that moves the eye to the left to fix the new object in the left temporal field which is then held in gaze and followed by either occipital lobe's pursuit system. The quick phase of this nystagmus is back towards its primary position.

Method of testing

The examiner utilizes a soft, wide cloth with 7.6 cm red blocks spaced 5 cm apart. The red blocks have to be wide to overcome any central fixation deficit. The tape is moved in all planes of gaze and the patient is asked to count the red blocks as they slip through the examiner's fingers.

The exact anatomic location of the occipital lobe pursuit and fixation centers as well as the fiber tracts that mediate supranuclear control of conjugate gaze is not known, but the fiber efferents are believed to lie anteriorly in the internal capsule and thalamus.

The test is useful for detecting parietal lobe lesions, distinguishing between the causes of an occipital lobe lesion, and to evaluate better adduction lag in a patient with an internuclear ophthalmoplegia. Any deep parietal lobe lesion will interrupt fibers from the occipital lobe pursuit system to the ipsilateral FEFs so that targets moving towards the side of the lesion can be tracked to the edge of the visual fields, but new targets appearing in the contralateral field cannot be fixed. The eyes stay to the side of the lesion. If the lesion is in the occipital lobe alone and there is no edema that might disrupt parietal lobe integrity, it is most likely an infarction. The normal other occipital lobe can effect pursuit. If, on the other hand, the occipital lobe lesion causes edema, the parietal lobe of the affected side will be compromised and the eyes will remain deviated to the side of the lesion

46

(Cogan's law). MRI evaluation has made this part of the examination less important. If the examiner wishes to stress the medial rectus muscle in a possible internuclear ophthalmoplegia, the examiner turns the head laterally to the side of the affected muscle and then asks the patient to follow the tape from lateral to medial. This maneuver makes it easier to uncover a partial intranuclear ophthalmoplegia. MRI scans rarely demonstrate the subtle lesions of the MLF that are causative of an intranuclear opthalmoplegia. If opticokinetic nystagmus is obtainable, the patient is not blind as he or she must be able to fix on a moving block of the tape.

Fifth cranial nerve

Anatomy

The nerve has a major sensory portion, motor component and three associated nuclei: the rostral, interpolaris and caudal nuclei. It carries all modalities of sensation from the face, the anterior part of the scalp, the eye and somatic sensation from the anterior two-thirds of the tongue. It also innervates the gum, teeth, mucous membranes of the cheeks, nasal passages, sinuses and the anterior components of the palate and nasopharynx. It is the motor innervation of the masseter, medial and lateral pterygoids, the tensor veli palatini and the anterior belly of the digastric and mylohyoid muscles.

The sensory divisions are extremely important in the diagnosis of head and neck pain. Difficulty occurs when its major divisions overlap with the innervation of the cervical plexus (posterior roots of C2–C4) from which is derived the pre- and postauricular nerve, seventh nerve innervation to the mastoid and external auditory canal, dural projections from C2, and a meningeal branch (sixth nerve) which innervates the tentorium.

Methods of examination

Superficial skin sensation

The major innervation zones of the fifth nerve are easily tested with the cold of the tuning fork (for A-delta fiber sensation), a cotton wisp for light touch (8–10 μm fibers) and a pin for C fiber (1 μm) burning pain.

The forehead and upper part of the side of the nose comprise the ophthalmic division V_1. This is the division that is tested by the corneal reflex. The corneal reflex can also be tested by placing a cotton applicator stick in the nose to the level of the orbit. This elicits a sneeze (the sternutatory reflex). This reflex can be used if the patient has a desensitized cornea (environmental desensitization ophthalmic surgery). The malar region and the upper lips are the core zones of the maxillary division; the chin lower jaw and anterior two-thirds of the tongue (ability of the patient to feel touch, not taste) is the core of the mandibular division.

Variable innervations

1 On the scalp the fifth nerve innervation does not stop at the hairline, but overlaps with C2, 2.5–5 cm from the vertex of the skull.

2 The mandibular supply to the pinna always includes the tragus. It may also innervate a strip along the upper and anterior margin of the pinna. Here it overlaps with the preauricular nerve from the posterior roots of C2–C3.

3 The angle of the jaw is supplied by cervical segment (C2).

4 The brainstem anatomy of the fifth nerve sensory division is complicated, but if mastered is extremely helpful in localization of lesions. All modalities of sensation from the nerve project to the Gasserian ganglia (Meckel's cave at the petrous apex). Fibers subserving touch synapse in the nucleus in the pons, cross the midline and ascend to synapse in the ventroposteromedial thalamic nucleus. Pain and temperature fibers synapse with the main sensory medius as it descends to C2 in the cord. The ophthalmic division may descend as low as T2. These fibers all cross the midline (quintothalamic tract) to synapse in the ventroposterior medial nucleus (VPM) of the thalamus. The face is inverted in the descending spinothalamic tract such that a lesion at cervical levels may cause numbness of the forehead. This is an excellent point when examining patients who have had neck trauma or if a syrinx is suspected. Remember that a subtle Horner's syndrome may be present as sympathetic fibers that supply the tarsal plates of the eyelids synapse at C8–T1 (ciliary center of Budge).

Abnormalities of sensation

Total loss of sensation over the entire distribution of the three divisions

This requires a lesion of the ganglion or an extension of a lesion anterior to the ganglion that involves all divisions. If this occurs, the motor root is involved. The usual causes of a complete fifth nerve lesion are metastatic, skull-based tumors, schwannomas, meningiomas and epidermoids that originate in the cerebellopontine angle, a neurofibroma of the nerve itself and meningeal processes such as syphilis or sarcoid. Rarely, chemotherapeutic agents, Sjögren's syndrome, paraneoplastic processes and scleroderma affect the nerve selectively. Stilbamidine (used for blastomycosis) and trichloroethylene (refrigerant) may involve the nerve. There is a probable autoimmune form of trigeminal sensory neuropathy. If the sensory loss in the face is complete and is associated with similar hemisensory loss, the lesion is in the contralateral thalamus or, rarely, the brainstem.

Total sensory loss over one or more divisions

This is seen most commonly with partial lesions of the ganglion (herpes zoster or of a root from compression of a cerebellopontine angle tumor).

The ophthalmic division is involved in the cavernous sinus along with the third, fourth and sixth nerve by a carotid aneurysm. The sixth nerve is next to the carotid artery in the sinus and is also involved by tumors in the superior orbital fissure. The maxillary division is involved by tumors and granulomatous processes at the posterior portion of the cavernous sinus. If involved solely, it is usually traumatic. Skull-based tumors involve both the sensory and motor root.

Isolated loss of touch

Touch fibers synapse in the pons. Touch loss alone is most often a basilar branch arterial lesion, demyelinating disease, pontine tumor or compression by brainstem displacement.

Pain and temperature loss with preservation of touch

This occurs from a lesion of the descending tract or nucleus in the medulla. The most common cause is infarction of the posterior inferior cerebellar artery. Most often the parent vertebral artery is infarcted. Patients complain of an ipsilateral "salt and pepper" painful facial sensation. The ascending spinothalamic tract is infarcted concomitantly and patients lose sensation to pain and temperature below the clavicle contralaterally. Other causes of this dissociation are syringobulbia, foramen magnum tumors, platybasia, basilar invagination and, rarely, demyelinating disease. Rarely, a high cervical lesion can cause loss of pain and temperature in the ophthalmic division (forehead).

Hyperesthesias over all or partial root distributions

Usually this is an irritative rather than a destructive lesion. It is most common in vascular lesions and herpes zoster and least common in syringobulbia. The most common mistake in evaluating the fifth nerve is confusion with the radiations of the preauricular nerve (posterior roots of C2–C3) that are sensitized with cervical plexus injury. The injury of these roots occurs concomitantly with injury of the roots and divisions of the brachial plexus (whiplash injury). The core zone of innervations of the nerve is the cheek, eye and mandible. It is most often confused with tic douloureux. The trigger zones for tic (initiated by a light touch) are:

1 corner of the upper lip;
2 alae of the nose;
3 temporomandibular joint;
4 below the lower lip.

These triggers are frequently in the same distribution as a cat's whiskers. A moving light touch often elicits the tic more readily than a static stimulus. Tic pain rarely lasts more than 10 seconds, is lancinating and very severe. Preauricular nerve pain is dull and may last for hours, days or weeks.

Corneal reflex

The innervation of the cornea is complicated. Nerve V_1 innervates the top one-third, there is a neutral zone in the middle and V_2 possibly innervates the lower one-third. Alternatively, the entire cornea may be innervated by V_1. The examiner has the patient look up and touches the top of the cornea with a wisp of cotton. Those patients who are skittish about any object approaching their eyes may be tested by blowing a little breath on the eye that is tested while shielding the other eye. The seventh nerve is the efferent arc of the reflex, and normally stimulating either cornea initiates a bilateral blink. If the cornea is stimulated and there is no response, the defect can be on either the afferent (sixth side) or the efferent seventh nerve side of the reflex arc. If there is a fifth nerve lesion, there will be a blink of both eyes when the normal side is stimulated and no response in either eye when the affected side is stimulated (afferent defect). If the seventh nerve is involved there will be no response if either side is stimulated. There will be a blink response of the normal side when the abnormal side is stimulated.

Loss of the corneal reflex is very helpful in localizing a peripheral fifth nerve lesion. It may be the first sign of a cerebellar pontine angle (CPA) tumor (the nerve exits the mid pons and turns north to enter the cavernous sinus) and may be involved along this course. Alternatively, an extra-canalicular eighth nerve schwannoma may compress the lateral pons and damage the descending tract of ophthalmic fibers. It is also very important in accessing brainstem function in comatose patients. Stimulating the cornea on one side initiates jaw deviation contralaterally. The corneal reflex is also important in relation to cavernous sinus aneurysms and tumors as well as disease of the superior orbital fissure.

Some patients have insensitive corneas. This is prevalent in those who have constant wind stimulation to their face and with exophthalmos. Patients may not be able to tell subjective sensory differences.

The preauricular nerve, from the cervical plexus (posterior roots of C2–C3) also projects into the face. If this nerve is irritated, patients frequently demonstrate neurogenic edema (hyperemia, edema, and heat on much of the face). Allodynia and hyperalgesia to pinprick as well as cold-induced nociceptive pain may be noted. This problem is commonly confused with lesions of the fifth nerve.

In Bell's palsy, patients frequently have decreased sensitivity of the face. This may be caused by concomitant involvement of the fifth nerve (autoimmune process) or from disturbance of sensorimotor integration of the fifth nerve at higher levels. The seventh nerve is supposed to be exclusively motor except for the external auditory canal or mastoid bone.

Patients who simulate fifth nerve sensory loss seldom are aware that fifth nerve innervation extends beyond the hairline and that C2 usually covers the angle of the jaw.

Bilateral loss of pain and temperature in the mid face implies a lesion of the medial medulla at the decussation of the ventrotegmental tract. It was fairly common in the past from trigeminal entry zone pathology from syphilis.

Motor function

The muscles of mastication are the temporal, masseter and pterygoids. The pterygoids move the jaws from side to side while chewing and the masseter and temporal muscles clench the jaws. Placing the fingers lightly on the masseter muscle and then asking the patient to bite down tests the latency of contraction and its force. As the jaws are opened they are pushed forward. The opposing pterygoids are balanced. If one is weak, the jaw deviates to the side of the weak muscle. If the lesion is supranuclear (corticobulbar fibers are lesioned), the jaw will deviate to the opposite side. The symmetry of the temporal fossa and the angles of the jaw should be noted. The examiner places his or her hand against the side of the jaw and instructs the patient to push against it. Ipsilateral weakness or deviation occurs from a contralateral supranuclear lesion or an ipsilateral nuclear lesion. The ability to swallow without choking is accomplished by the tensor veli palatini muscle which closes off the nasopharynx. Lower motor pathologies such as motor neuron disease or tumor are associated with hollowing at the temple and flattening of the angle of the jaw. Intermittent weakness of the muscles of mastication occurs with myasthenia gravis, giant cell arteritis (claudication of mastication), Takayasu's disease, and rarely with branchial myopathy in which the muscles may swell with chewing. It has rarely been seen with the Lambert–Eaton syndrome (paraneoplastic).

Jaw jerk (Fig. 3.10)

The jaw jerk is helpful in localization in the brainstem and, in conjunction with other reflexes, gives information in regard to the patient's reflex status. It is dependent on the mesencephalic tract of the fifth cranial nerve which mediates proprioceptive information from jaw muscles. The patient is instructed to open the jaw slightly and the examiner places a forefinger below the lower lip and gently taps it downward with the reflex hammer. There is a slightly palpable upward movement. It is frequently unobtainable in normal people.

Abnormalities

In supranuclear lesions that are above the mid pons, the jaw jerk is uninhibited (exactly similar to an exaggerated knee jerk) and is increased at times to clonus. This is seen in neurodegenerative diseases with generalized loss of cortical inhibition, pseudobulbar palsy (bilateral damage of corticobulbar projections), motor neuron disease and multiple sclerosis.

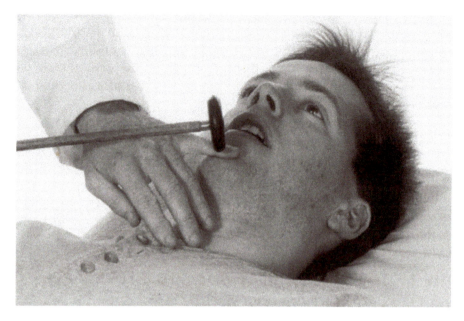

Fig. 3.10 The jaw jerk. A gentle tap is essential or the mechanical effect of the percussion will confuse the responses.

Trophic changes

Rarely, following trigeminal ganglia destruction from ablative procedures or autoimmune processes, there is erosion of the nasal alae and skin of the mid face. Midline granuloma can cause similar features that, if severe, cause corneal ulceration, infection and panophthalmitis. The seventh nerve maybe concomitantly involved, which compounds the problem as the patient is unable to constrict the orbicularis oculi and protect the cornea.

Seventh cranial nerve (Figs 3.11 & 3.12)

The facial nerve (seventh cranial nerve) and the nervus intermedius have a close anatomic relationship and are discussed together. The seventh nerve exits the lower one-third of the pons to enter the CPA and thence the internal auditory canal (IAC). It is superior to the eighth nerve in the IAC. It then traverses the petrous portion of the temporal bone in a horizontal and then vertical pathway to exit behind the stylomastoid process through the stylomastoid foramen.

The major motor functions are the innervations of the muscles of facial expression and movement, the superficial platysma muscle of the neck and the stapedius muscle of the ear.

The nervus intermedius carries afferent secretory fibers to the lacrimal glands through the greater superficial petrosal nerve and to the salivary glands through the chorda tympani which mediates taste for the anterior two-thirds of the tongue.

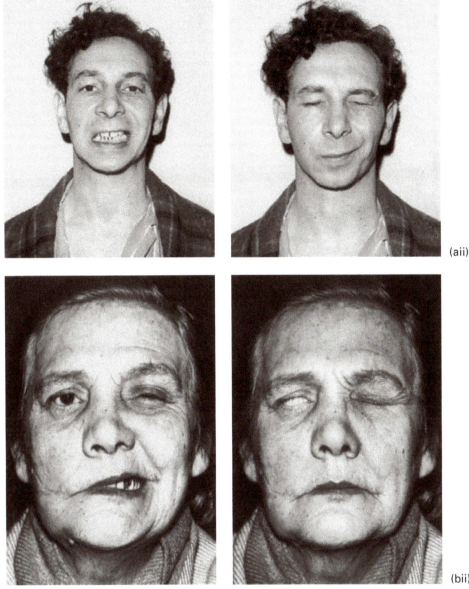

(ai)

(aii)

(bi)

(bii)

Fig. 3.11 (a) Upper motor neuron facial paresis. (ai) The weakness of the lower part of the face is very much greater than the upper. (aii) In this case associated movements of the right lower facial muscles were also affected. (b) Lower motor neuron facial paralysis. Both upper and lower parts of the face are equally involved. Note absence of wrinkling or right forehead and visible sclera on screwing up eyes. (*Cont'd on page 54*).

Methods of examination

Inspection

1   The symmetry of the face.
2   The wrinkles of the forehead and the prominence or flatness of the nasolabial folds.

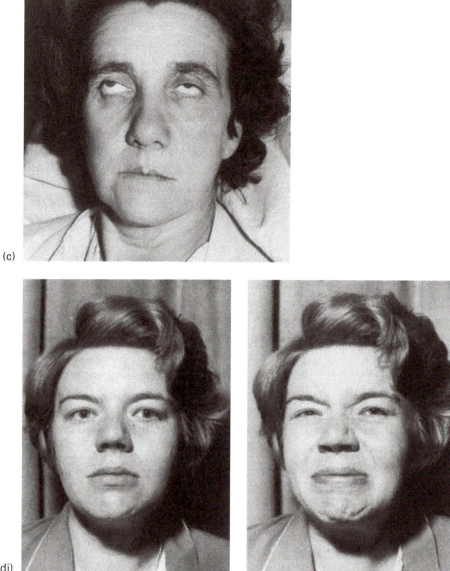

(c)

(di)

(dii)

Fig. 3.11 (*cont'd*) (c) Bilateral lower motor neuron facial paralysis. The patient is trying to close her eyes. The eyeballs move upwards, but are uncovered; the lower part of the face is flattened and expressionless. (d) Old bilateral lower motor neuron facial paralysis with aberrant reinnervation: (di) at rest; (dii) on smiling.

3 The symmetry of blinking; the eyeballs should turn up and out with each blink. This is a normal phenomenon but is not seen because of full closure of the lids if there is no weakness.

4 Spontaneous movements of the mouth. Note abnormal movements such as twitching, tremor, involuntary movements and myokymia. This is a vermicular (worm-like) undulating movement around the eye which may be associated with a pontine glioma or demyelinating disease. Hemifacial

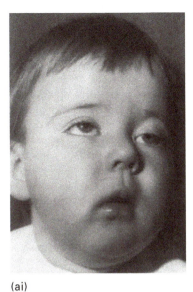
(ai)

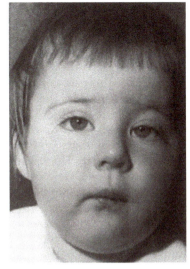
(aii)

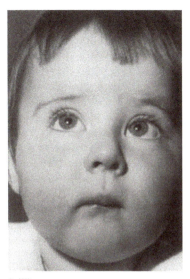
(aiii)

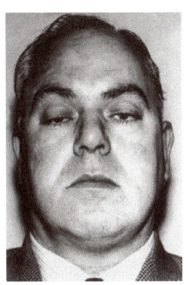
(bi)

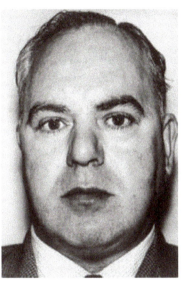
(bii)

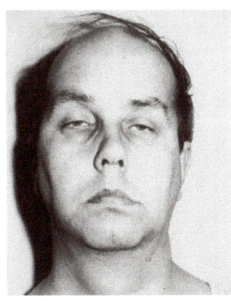
(c)

Fig. 3.12 (a) Effects of neostigmine on myasthenia gravis: (ai) before injection; (aii) 10 minutes after injection; and (aiii) 20 minutes after injection. These photographs are intended also as a reminder that this disease can affect the very young. (b) Effects of edrophonium chloride (Tensilon) on myasthenia gravis: (bi) before injection; and (bii) 60 seconds after injection. (c) Myotonic dystrophy. Baldness, ptosis, myopathic facies and absence of sternomastoids.

spasm and oculopalatal myoclonus (rhythmic movement of the platysma muscle in conjunction with the palate) are quite specific. In the former, there is an abnormal branch of the anterior inferior cerebellar artery impinging on the seventh nerve and in the latter a lesion (usually vascular) in Mollaret's triangle. These are connections between the red nucleus, dentate and inferior olivary nucleus.

Motor functions

The examiner asks the patient to mimic him or her in baring the teeth. Note the symmetry of the movement with particular attention to the nasolabial folds. Ask the patient to open the mouth and note the symmetry of the nasolabial folds. The upper facial muscles are tested by asking the patient to close the eyes tightly and to resist the examiner opening them. The patient is then asked to frown, wrinkle the forehead and raise the eyebrows. Weakness of facial muscles is apparent as asymmetry. The platysma is tested by having the patient bare the teeth and open the mouth simultaneously. Blowing out the cheeks and pursing the lips tests the lower facial muscles.

Examination of taste

There are four primary tastes:
1 Sweet
2 Sour
3 Salt
4 Bitter

All others are flavors and depend on an intact sense of smell.

The patient is asked to protrude the tongue to the side. The tip is gently held with a piece of gauze. The patient points to a card on which the four possible tastes are written. The side of the tongue is moistened with the test substances 2 cm from its tip. The patient swishes out the mouth with water between applications of the test substances which are sugar, salt, vinegar and quinine. A qualitative assessment of taste is now performed with electrical depolarization of taste buds (produces a metallic taste) in taste and smell centers.

Secretory functions

Schirmer's test is performed by gently applying a strip of filter paper from the lower eyelids and measuring the length of moistening on each side after the patient is stimulated to tear by inhaling ammonia. This is helpful in Sjögren's syndrome. Saliva flow is rarely tested. If the examiner stimulates its flow by placing a spicy substance on the tongue, which is slightly raised, the examiner can compare submaxillary flow from side to side.

Types of facial weakness

Unilateral facial paralysis

The facial nerve has two major innervations. The cortical innervation derives from area 4 of the motor cortex and is bilateral to the upper facial muscles. The degree of the bilateral innervation varies from person to person. The seventh nerve nucleus is also innervated from the contralateral basal ganglia, thalamus and temporal lobe. This innervation and its projection to the frontal lobe constitute the "mimetic" or "emotional facial." It is responsible for the normal play of facial expression during speech and with laughter. If a patient laughs spontaneously, the facial muscles opposite a lesion (of the thalamus, basal ganglia or temporal lobe) do not contract. If the patient is asked to voluntarily smile, these muscles contract.

An upper motor facial paralysis occurs from a lesion of the motor cortex (the facial component of the homunculus) or its projections to the facial nerve nucleus in the lateral lower one-third of the pons. The orbicularis oris, buccinator and risus sardonicus muscles of the lower facial musculature will not contract and the nasolabial fold will be flat. The upper facial muscles will contract because of their bilateral innervation. An associated hemiplegia will be on the same side as the facial weakness and a concomitant hemianopsia places it in the hemisphere above the tentorium.

In a lower motor neuron weakness, both the upper and lower facial muscles are involved. The eye musculature is weak, the eye turns upward on attempted closure, and the patient is unable to blink or wrinkle the forehead on the side of the lesion. This occurs because the final common pathway between the seventh nerve nucleus and the muscles it innervates is interrupted. The associated signs and symptoms determine if the lesion is near the nucleus or more peripheral as the motor fibers innervate their individual muscles.

Sites of a unilateral lower motor neuron weakness of the seventh nerve

If the sixth nerve is involved, the lesion is in the pons as the seventh nerve fibers wrap around the sixth nerve nucleus before they exit laterally. If the fifth and eighth nerve are involved, the lesion is in the CPA. It is usually a tumor with consequent ipsilateral ataxia and contralateral weakness. Rotary nystagmus more prominent to the side of the lesion is noted.

If taste, salivation and lacrimation are involved the lesion lies close to the brainstem prior to the bifurcation of the chorda tympani in the middle ear. The stapedius muscle is affected at this level and sounds are distorted and too loud. If taste and salivation are affected, but lacrimation is normal, the lesion is in the middle ear between the superficial petrosal nerve and the chorda tympani.

If only motor weakness of the nerve is determined, the lesion is usually in the facial canal peripheral to the take off of the chorda tympani. Rarely, it is in the nucleus itself. If only some of the facial muscles are involved, particularly those innervating the upper face, the process is usually in the parotid gland or the muscles themselves. Perineural spread of salivary gland tumors (mixed adenocarcinomas or cylindromas, "sugar-coated nerve tumors") as well as squamous cell carcinoma of the skin or the infratemporal fossa gradually produce lower motor neuron facial weakness by infiltrating the nerve.

Bilateral facial weakness

This is often missed because there is apparent facial symmetry.

Bilateral mimetic or emotional facial palsy occurs with Parkinson's and other basal ganglia syndromes. The patient blinks less than seven times per minute (when it occurs it is normal). The face is mask-like and there is little emotional play. The face becomes normal when the patient smiles.

The characteristics of bilateral upper motor neuron lesions (pseudobulbar palsy) between the cortex and the seventh nerve nucleus are as follow:
1 blinking is normal;
2 there is less masked facies;
3 the mouth cannot move on command, but appears to move normally spontaneously.
It is usually associated with other cranial nerve abnormalities (hyperactive jaw jerk), spastic dysarthria and generalized spasticity.

Bilateral lower motor neuron palsy causes a transverse smile, sagging of the corners of the mouth in repose, flattening of the nasal labial folds and fewer forehead wrinkles. The patient is unable to effect voluntary facial movement and the white of the eyes are evident on blink or eye closure. The patient has a labial dysarthria (cannot pronounce Methodist Episcopal, particularly Episcopal).

Aberrant regeneration

Following peripheral facial denervation there is often abnormal reinnervation. This is manifest as "jaw winking" (the patient opens the mouth and there is ptosis of the affected eye), gustatory sweating in which eating causes hyperhidrosis of the face, and spontaneous twitching of specific muscles. Perhaps the most common sign of aberrant reinnervation is mentalis muscle of the chin contracture with eye closure. If there is bilateral aberrant innervation, the entire face may contract with an expression that may be inappropriate for the expressed emotion.

Primary muscle disorders and anterior horn cell disease

In myasthenia gravis, all facial muscles are weak. There is concomitant ptosis and extraocular paresis (Fig. 3.13). There is markedly decreased facial expression and a transverse smile (weakness of the risus sardonicus

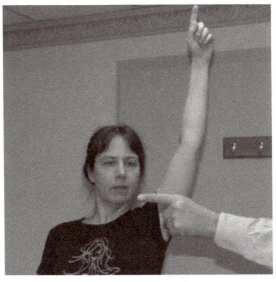

(a)

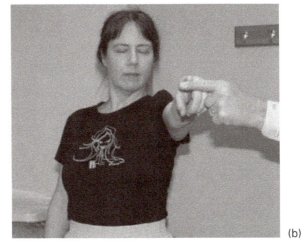

(b)

Fig. 3.13 Past pointing cerebellar versus vestibular cause. (a) The patient is instructed to touch the outstretched finger of the examiner with the eyes closed. (b) Normal accurate response. (c) The patient past points to the side of the lesion with cerebellar disease. In this instance, it would be to the left. (*Cont'd on page 60*).

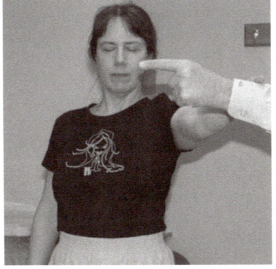

(c)

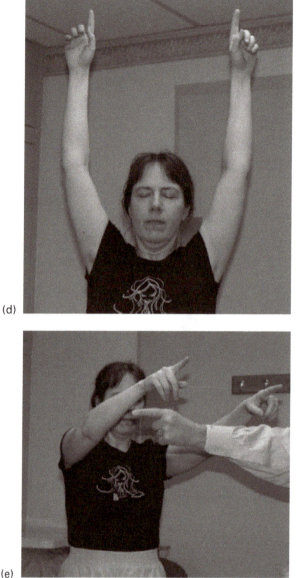

(d)

(e)

Fig. 3.13 (*cont'd*) (d) Both arms past point to the left with a left vestibular lesion. (e) The right vestibular system predominates and innervates both sides of the body.

peripheral perioral muscles) so that the corners of the mouth do not contract.

In oculopharyngeal dystrophy, fascioscapulo humeral dystrophy (FSHD), mitochondrial myopathies, some congenital myopathies (nemaline) and rarely somatic muscular atrophy (SMA) (Kennedy's syndrome) and bulbar neuronopathy there is bilateral weakness of facial muscles. Characteristic of Kennedy's syndrome are facial fasciculations and enlarged breasts in men (mutation of androgen receptor). Myotonic dystrophy demonstrates a classic myopathic facies (see Fig. 3.13). These patients have atrophy of the temporalis muscles with hollowing, loss of masseter muscle bulk and bilateral ptosis. They have a "hatchet jaw" appearance. On first glance these patients have a long, thin and expressionless face. There are downward lines at the corner of the eyes and mouth and a transverse smile as is also noted with myasthenia gravis. In myotonic dystrophy, forced eye closure maybe associated with inability to open them quickly. This form of localized myotonia is frequently exacerbated by a cold cloth over the eyes. It is less severe in congenital myotonias.

Vestibular nerve (see Fig. 3.13)

Displacement of hair cells in the ampullae of the semicircular canals and the otoliths of the sacculus and utriclus by endolymph depolarize mechanoreceptive receptors (sodium channels) of the vestibular nerve to generate impulses. The nerve projects to the vestibular ganglia and then to the vestibular nuclei of the medulla. The connections of the vestibular nerve are widespread. They project to the oculomotor nuclei through the medial longitudinal fasciculus, many regions of the cerebellum – the most important of which is the floccular nodular lobe – and to the upper cervical segments of the spinal cord. Projections to the nucleus tractus solitarius (NTS) mediate brainstem reflexes which include nausea, vomiting and hyperhidrosis. The perception of vertigo, formerly thought to be in the superior temporal gyrus, has now moved to the intraparietal sulcus. The lateral vestibular nucleus of Deiters is the origin of the lateral vestibular spinal tract and consequently is important for motor functions of the vestibular nerve.

Examination of hearing

Place a finger in the external auditory meatus opposite the ear to be tested and move it continuously to produce a masking sound. Ask the patient to repeat "26" or "68" whispered into the tested ear to test high tones and "42" or "100" to test low tones. The examiner must use the otoscope to be certain there is no pathology of the middle ear and eardrum that would block sound transmission.

Type of deafness

Rinne's test

The tuning fork is gently struck, mask the contralateral ear and hold it near the external auditory meatus of the tested ear. If the patient can hear it, move it to the mastoid bone. The second the patient can no longer hear it ask him or her to say "now." Then hold it near the external auditory meatus and ask if he or she can still hear it. In a normal patient the sound is still audible. In deafness, from middle ear disease, the patient will not be able to hear the vibration. In incomplete nerve deafness both air and bone conduction are decreased, but air conduction may still be perceived.

Weber's test

The vibrating tuning fork is placed in the middle of the forehead, and then ask the patient where he or she hears it. In nerve deafness, the patient perceives the sound in the normal ear, whereas in chronic middle ear disease, it is heard in the affected ear.

Common causes of nerve (perceptual) deafness

1 *At the cochlear level.* Ménière's disease (high frequency loss that is often bilateral), otosclerosis, prolonged exposure to loud noise; internal auditory artery occlusion.

2 *At the eighth nerve level.* Cerebellar pontine angle tumors (schwannoma, meningioma and epidermoid), trauma, surgery, postinflammatory lesions, siderosis (iron deposition from past multiple intracranial hemorrhages), post-inflammatory conditions (meningitis), toxins, autoimmune diseases, multiple syndromic and hereditary familial diseases.

3 *In the brainstem.* There are rare vascular malformations, demyelinating events, tumors or central pontine myelinolysis that affect hearing at this level. Detecting the cause of deafness cannot be performed at the bedside in this instance and requires the use of MRI and thin slice CT (rules out structural lesions), pure tone audiometry, speech discrimination, loudness recruitment, tone decay and Békésy audiometry.

In general, middle ear deafness has loss of low tones and nerve deafness loss of high tones. Loudness recruitment occurs with lesions of the hair cells of the organ of Corti and is most often seen in Ménière's disease and otosclerosis rather than retrocochlear pathologies. Tone decay is more suggestive of an eighth nerve tumor rather than a cochlear lesion. If the intensity has to be raised by greater than 20 dB in less than 3 minutes, a tumor of the eighth nerve is likely.

Acoustic reflex testing is very sensitive for middle ear and ossicle disease. Electrocochleography can distinguish different forms of sensorineural hearing loss.

Clinical examination of vestibular function

Disturbance of vestibular function causes falling, past pointing, vertigo and nystagmus. As with tests of auditory functions, the examiner can make an educated guess as to the side of the difficulty and the circumstances of its occurrence and thus narrow the diagnostic possibilities. The easiest way to evaluate vestibular function is to utilize the hands as for conjugate gaze centers. Flex the hands so that the fingers of the left hand are pointing to the right hand. Thus, if there is a lesion of the right vestibular system the left will be predominant and the patient will past point to the left, fall to the left and drift on pendular walking to the left. The cortex will correct for the eyes being driven to the left and the fast component of corrective nystagmus will be to the right.

Pendular walking (Fig. 3.14)

The patient is instructed to go to the corner of the room, close the eyes and walk in a straight line, back and forth. The examiner explains to the patient that he or she will be stopped before crashing into an object. The second the patient closes the eyes he or she broadens their stance. During the maneuver the patient drifts to the side of the lesion as the opposite vestibular complex predominates.

Past pointing (see Fig. 3.14)

The patient is seated in front of the examiner and asked to close the hand except for the index finger. The patient is instructed to raise and lower the finger to touch the outstretched finger of the examiner. The patient is then instructed to perform the maneuver rapidly. The patient will past point with both hands to the side of the lesion. If the patient has a cerebellar lesion, he or she will past point with the hand on the side of the cerebellar lesion while the other hand remains on target. The examiner will not see dramatic changes in chronic disease. Acutely, the patient is often too ill to perform the maneuver. Patients with vestibular disease feel as if they are

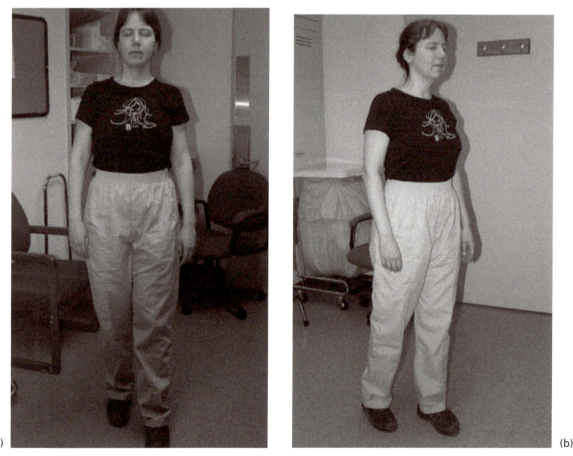

(a)

(b)

Fig. 3.14 Pendular walking. (a) The examiner instructs the patient to walk backwards and forwards with the eyes closed. Most patients do this extremely accurately.
(b) The patient drifts to the left. The left vestibular system is deficient and the right side predominates. The patient will fall to the left with the eyes closed and will past point to the left. The patient broadens her base.

pushed to the affected side. Patients with cerebellar lesions fall to the affected side as they are clumsy with the affected foot. Utricular and saccular disease may cause the patient to be pushed in a linear direction. Vestibular sensations of dramatic displacement are termed pulsions. Thus, a patient who has acute loss of vestibular function on the left side may feel as if he or she is pushed to the left and would have lateral pulsion. This is not uncommon in a posterior inferior cerebellar artery (PICA) stroke.

Caloric tests

This test is used in comatose patients. Because there are no corrective responses (the cortex is non-functional), the eyes will deviate to the side of the lesion. The patient is placed 30° above horizontal. Cold water at 30° (100 mL; some say 1 mL) is irrigated through a soft rubber catheter for 40 seconds into the right external auditory meatus. The eyes deviate to the side of the irrigated ear. If the right vestibular system is working, the eyes stay deviated for 30 seconds to 1 minute and then return to the midline. The test is repeated in the other ear and if the eyes conjugately deviate, the vestibular system, the extraocular muscles and the MLF are intact. It is best to think of the cold water as shutting off the stimulated vestibular system. In fact, raising the head 30° from the horizontal position places the ampulla that will be stimulated in the vertical plane with the ampulla being at the highest point. Warm water will cause the endolymph to rise and stimulate the canal to drive the eyes to the right. Cold water will cause the endolymph to flow in the downward direction, which would generate less stimulation to the ipsilateral ear and the eyes would be driven to the side of the infused cold water stimulation because the endolymph would flow away from the cold stimulated ear. It is easier to think of the test as cold water shutting down the irrigated ear.

Canal paresis is the term used to describe an absent or diminished caloric test. This is usually caused by a lesion of the labyrinth such as Ménière's disease, an acoustic tumor, vestibular neuronitis or autoimmune etiologies. MRI with gadolinium enhancement demonstrates tumors (often the specific type) and inflammatory conditions. Thin cut CT radiography demonstrates bony erosion and fractures. It is rare to need caloric testing in the modern age of neuroimaging. Magnetic resonance angiography can demonstrate an aberrant branch of the anterior inferior cerebellar artery (brought to neurologic attention by Dr. Janetta's observations of its occurrence with tic douloureux), which impinges upon the eighth nerve and diminishes its function.

Positional vertigo and nystagmus

The patient lies on the examination table with the shoulders at the cephalad edge of the table. The examiner lowers the head 30° and turns it to the side. Patients with positional vertigo will develop vertigo, usually within 10–15 seconds, associated with nystagmus, the fast component of which beats toward the down ear. Adaptation occurs and the symptoms and signs cannot be reproduced for 10–15 minutes. This may be because of utricular lesions although it has recently been reported from posterior semicircular canal (PCC) disease. It is seen from degeneration of the cupula (cupulolithiasis) vascular lesions and head trauma. It occurs most frequently when arising from sleep.

Central positional vertigo is most often caused by a tumor of the posterior fossa and is characterized by:

1 no latency;

2 no adaptation;

3 the nystagmus appears immediately when the former provoking position is resumed.

The nystagmus will change direction with different head positions.

Patients with positional nystagmus from central lesions often have positional vertigo with movement, but it is more prolonged and severe. It usually is associated with other long tract or cerebellar signs.

Common vestibular pathologies

Labyrinth. Ménière's disease, motion sickness, drug toxicity (hair cell destruction by the mycin antibiotics and migraine (there is a malignant form with severe vertigo).

Vestibular nerve. Schwannoma and other CPA tumors, trauma, autoimmune disorders, syphilis, hypothyroidism, an aberrant branch of anterior inferior cerebellar artery (AICA) compression, low pressure headache (traction on the nerve) and vestibular neuronitis (viral origin).

In the brainstem. Vertebrobasilar insufficiency (older patients), cerebellar and fourth ventricular tumors, demyelinating and other acute autoimmune diseases (acute disseminated encephalomyelitis, acute hemorrhagic leukoencephalopathy), migraine are causative in the brainstem.

At the cortical level, the temporal lobe and intraparietal gyrus are involved. The usual pathologies are complex partial seizures, vascular disease, herpes simplex, migraine and trauma.

Ninth and tenth cranial nerves

Clinically and anatomically it is difficult to separate the glossopharyngeal and vagus (ninth and tenth cranial nerves) so they are discussed together.

The most important functions of the vagus and glossopharyngeal nerves in neurologic practice are as follow:

1 Somatic sensation from the pharynx, larynx, tonsils, soft palate and posterior one-third of the tongue

2 The sense of taste from the posterior one-third of the tongue (primarily the ninth nerve)

3 The motor innervation of the palate and pharyngeal muscles

4 The motor innervation of the vocal cords (tenth nerve)

5 Cardiovascular, respiratory and gastrointestinal reflexes (ninth and tenth nerves)

Methods of examination

Initial observation

The examiner notes the pitch and quality of the patient's voice, spontaneous cough and the ability to swallow. Regurgitation of fluids is sought by history. A high-pitched hoarse voice suggests vocal cord paralysis, whereas a nasal tone that increases with forward flexion is characteristic of palate weakness. This improves with the head extended. If the patient chokes on saliva while speaking this is characteristic of both palatal and pharyngeal weakness. Myasthenia is suggested by worsening of symptomatology with fatigue (there is almost always associated ptosis and extraocular muscle dysfunction).

Motor function

The examiner asks the patient to open the mouth wide. The examiner inspects the uvula and the tongue while it is at rest on the floor of the mouth. A fibrillating tongue with scalloping at its edges (twelfth nerve) is most often motor neuron disease. The patient is asked to say "Ah" while exhaling and "Ugh" while inhaling. The palate should elevate and move backwards, the uvula remains in the midline while the posterior pharyngeal muscles contract. A deep breath alone elevates the palate and is easy for the patient to perform.

Sensory functions

Touch sensation

A throat swab is used to stimulate the back of the throat while the tongue is gently depressed. The sensory component of the gag reflex is elicited from any part of the palate, tonsil or posterior part of the tongue that is touched and initiates contraction of the pharynx (posterior constrictor muscles) elevation of the palate and tongue retraction. The threshold of the reflex varies from patient to patient.

Taste sensation

Testing taste in the posterior tongue is now primarily carried out in taste and smell centers. It is rarely necessary as pathology never affects this component of the nerve alone (possible exception is Hencken's syndrome type II).

Abnormalities

1   The uvula is pointed to one side. This is often apparent in normal people. If there is no lesion it moves normally with phonation.

2   Swelling in the tonsillar region. In neurologic practice this indicates carcinoma of the tonsil and nasopharynx or lymphoma. In the era of HIV it may be *Candida* infection (thrush).

3   Unilateral muscle paralysis.

4   Abnormal movements. Palatal myoclonus resulting from a lesion of the central tegmental tract. This is a rhythmic vertical oscillation of the palate which at times is in conjunction movement with the eyes, larynx and diaphragm.

On phonation

If there is lower motor neuron weakness of the vagus, the palate elevates and moves to the normal side. This pulling movement resembles cloth being pulled over a table. Bilateral absence of movement of the palate and pharynx is accompanied by dysphagia, nasal regurgitation and nasal speech. This is usually secondary to bilateral medullary lesions (the nucleus ambiguous from a PICA infarction) or a bilateral upper motor lesion from pseudobulbar palsy. Pseudobulbar palsy is accompanied by a hyperactive gag reflex, bilateral spasticity and Babinski's sign in association with an abnormal affect (inappropriate crying or laughter). It is most commonly seen with severe vascular disease, demyelinating disease and head trauma. A combination of both upper and lower motor neuron disease may be seen in amyotrophic lateral sclerosis (ALS). Repeated phonation causes fatigue-ability in myasthenia gravis.

Sensory loss

Unilateral absence of the gag reflex is seen with isolated lesions of the ninth nerve that occur with schwannomas, glomus jugulare tumors, lymphoma or a surgical procedure. The normal side will trigger a full reflex. Phonation and direct inspection of the pharynx demonstrates unilateral muscle weakness as a cause of unilateral decrease of a gag reflex.

A combination of glossopharyngeal and vagus lesions causes the palate and posterior pharynx to pull to the normal side when stimulated. A bilateral motor and sensory deficit of the pharynx is most often secondary to a severe medullary vascular lesion or tumor. Descending branchiocervical Guillain–Barré syndrome does not affect pharyngeal sensation.

An upper motor neuron lesion from vascular disease causes inability to elevate the palate and constrict the pharynx on the side contralateral to the lesion (the pharynx pulls and the palate elevates to the normal side).

Examining the vocal cords

This examination is required in any patient who is hoarse or whenever it is suspected that there is a neurologic lesion responsible for palatopharyngeal weakness. The examination is performed by an otolaryngologist. The movements of the vocal cord during inspiration, expiration and phonation (the patient saying "Ah") are recorded. The cords abduct during inspiration and adduct during phonation.

Abnormalities of the vocal cords

In general, neurologic diseases produce unilateral abductor paralysis or total unilateral paralysis. In the former, the vocal cord remains in the midline at rest and with inspiration, but moves slightly toward the midline (normal side) with phonation. This is caused by a lesion of the recurrent laryngeal nerve from the vagus. With total paralysis, the cord lies in mid-abduction, but is pulled to the normal side with phonation. This is caused by a severe lesion of the vagus nerve. Both conditions cause hoarseness.

If there is bilateral total paralysis, both cords are in mid-abduction, are immobile and speech is not possible. This is a result of bilateral vagal nerve lesions. Bilateral abductor paralysis causes opposition of both cords that do not move with inspiration, which causes respiratory obstruction. This is caused by bilateral recurrent nerve lesions (Semon's law) or rarely by nuclear brainstem lesions.

Vocal cord position

1 Unilateral abductor paralysis
    (a) cord midline at rest
    (b) recurrent laryngeal nerve
2 Total unilateral paralysis
    (a) mid-abduction at rest
    (b) vagal nerve
3 Bilateral total paralysis
    (a) mid-abduction of both cords
    (b) bilateral vagus lesion
4 Bilateral abductor paralysis
    (a) adducted cords
    (b) bilateral recurrent laryngeal nerve lesion

Lesions of the glossopharyngeal and vagus nerves

1 Unilateral pure motor paralysis
    (a) poliomyelitis, diphtheria, botulism
    (b) Epstein–Barr virus infection
    (c) rarely, autoimmune disease

(d)   myasthenia gravis (pure pharyngeal form)

(e)   Charcot–Marie–Tooth disease type 4C

(f)   neuralgia amyotrophica

2   Unilateral sensory loss

(a)   extremely rare

(b)   putative virus or autoimmune

3   Unilateral motor paralysis and sensory loss

(a)   destruction of the nucleus ambiguous

(i)   PICA infarction (medial branch)

(ii)   syringobulbia (at the alar plate)

(b)   posterior fossa tumors (glomus jugulae; schwannoma, metastatic disease of the skull base)

(c)   vascular abnormalities (cavernous hemangioma and arteriovenous malformations)

(d)   platybasia, congenital stenosis of neuronal exit foramina; fibrous dysplasia

(e)   glandular enlargement at or below the jugular foramina

4   Bilateral upper motor neuron paralysis

(a)   pseudobulbar palsy (bilateral severe brainstem vascular disease)

(b)   ALS and primary lateral sclerosis (PLS)

(c)   advanced Parkinson's disease and other akinetic rigid syndromes (progressive supranuclear palsy and multiple system atrophy)

(d)   severe closed head trauma

5   Bilateral lower motor neuron paralysis

(a)   Kennedy's syndrome (mutation of the androgen receptor gene with gynecomastia; on chromosome 4; a bulbar neuropathy)

(b)   poliomyelitis

(c)   *Botulinum* toxin

(d)   ALS and its juvenile form (Fazio–Londe disease)

6   Fatigueable motor paralysis

(a)   myasthenia gravis

(b)   Lambert–Eaton syndrome (paraneoplastic syndrome)

7   Palatal myoclonus

(a)   vascular lesion of the central tegmental tract

Lesions of the recurrent laryngeal nerve

1   Unilateral. Mediastinal tumors (most often malignant thymoma, lung carcinoma, metastatic); thoracic aortic aneurysms; thyroid carcinoma and its consequent surgery; trauma.

2   Bilateral enlarged infected or lymphomatous cervical glands, trauma, thyroid malignancy.

Eleventh cranial nerve (Fig. 3.15)

The spinal component of the accessory (eleventh) cranial nerve is primarily

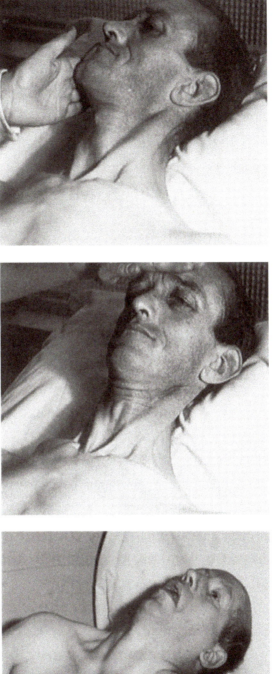

(a)

(b)

Fig. 3.15 Eleventh cranial nerve: the sternomastoids.
(a) Turning the head against resistance brings the opposite sternomastoid into action.
(b) Raising the head forwards against resistance brings both muscles into action.
(c) Typical result of bilateral sternomastoid weakness. On sitting up, the patient's head lags behind and overaction of platysma draws the mouth downwards.

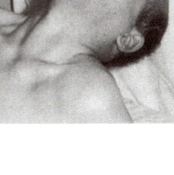

(c)

examined as it innervates the upper muscle fibers of the trapezius and the sternocleidomastoid muscles. It influences the posture and movement of the head and the shoulder girdle.

Methods of examination

Observation at rest

If the head is forward, trapezius weakness is suspected. The head falling backwards is indicative of sternocleidomastoid weakness. A dropped shoulder is often caused by trapezius and levator scapulae weakness.

Sternocleidomastoid tests

The patient sits and the examiner places his or her hand against the jaw. The patient is asked to turn the head against the examiner's hand. The opposite sternomastoid is seen to contract and is palpated. The patient is then asked to bend the head forward against the resistance of the examiner's hand which is placed against the forehead. Both sternomastoids will contract and can be compared. If the patient is lying flat in bed, he or she is asked to sit up and the examiner notes head movement (Fig. 3.16). In a normal person, the head leaves the pillow first and there is no lag or compensation by the platysma muscle.

Trapezius

Compare the line of the shoulder and the scapula. The medial scapular borders should be vertical and symmetrical. The examiner asks the patient to raise the shoulders toward the ears and tests this movement against resistance. At rest the scapula is displaced down and laterally.

Abnormalities

If there is sternomastoid wasting, the neck appears elongated, the muscles thin and the thyroid cartilage exaggerated. If there is bilateral weakness, there is severe difficulty in raising the head from the pillow. Unilateral weakness causes inability to turn the head to the opposite side. The muscle will not contract during this maneuver or with head flexion against resistance.

Trapezius weakness causes a dropped shoulder with lateral and downward displacement of the scapula. If the shoulder is also forward, the levator scapulae are involved. Raising the shoulder or shrugging against resistance is not completely absent because the lower component of the trapezius is innervated by the ventral roots of C1–C4 (cervical plexus).

Fasciculation of these muscles (trapezius and sternocleidomastoid) suggests a nuclear lesion or motor neuron disease. Irritative and compressive

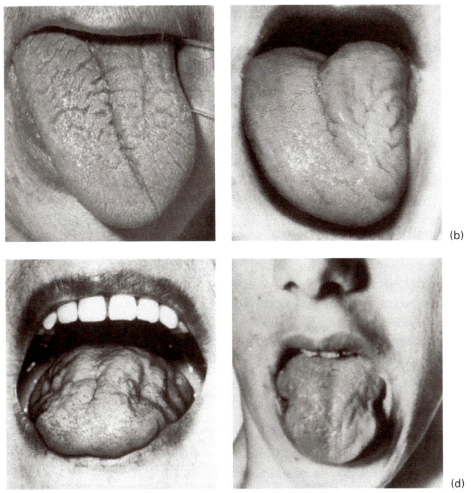

(a)

(b)

(c)

(d)

Fig. 3.16 Twelfth cranial nerve. (a) Early, and (b) advanced, left hypoglossal nerve palsy. Note reduction in size of affected side, excessive ridging and wrinkling, and curve of tip and median raphe towards the side of the lesion. (c) Bilateral wasting and spasticity in motor neuron disease. Note restricted protrusion, surface indentations and reduction in size without deviation. (d) Myotonia. Note characteristic prolonged dimpling after percussion of tongue.

lesions of the nerve trunk may also be associated with fasciculations and cervical dystonia.

Common lesions

1 *Bilateral sternomastoid paralysis.* Myotonic dystrophy, oculopharyngeal dystrophy, some congenital myopathies, motor neuron disease, spinal muscular atrophy and cervicobrachial descending GBS.

2 *A general rule for the sternomastoids.* Flexor weakness greater than extensor weakness suggests muscle disease. Extensor weakness greater than flexor weakness is motor neuron disease (dropped head syndrome). If both are equally weak, the problem is myasthenia gravis or a neuromuscular junction disease. The rule works approximately 50% of the time.

3 *Bilateral trapezius paralysis.* Motor neuron disease, scapuloperoneal dystrophies, hereditary sensory neuropathy type II, severe polyneuropathy and poliomyelitis. West Nile fever may give a similar poliomyelitis-like clinical picture.

Unilateral lesions

Trauma to the neck or the base of the skull; the accessory nerve is often injured with biopsy of lymph nodes in the posterior triangle of the neck; neurotropic viruses; hereditary sensory motor neuropathy (HSMN) type II (isolated muscle weakness); jugular foramen tumors (glomus jugulae, meningioma, schwannoma or skull-based metastasis); platybasia; syringomyelia with or without Chiari malformation.

Twelfth cranial nerve (see Fig. 3.16)

The hypoglossal nerve (twelfth) is a purely motor nerve and controls all movements of the tongue. It is also involved with specific movements of the hyoid bone and larynx during and following swallowing.

Method of examination

The patient is instructed to open the mouth and the tongue is evaluated for bulk, shape, position and its surfaces. At complete rest, if it is denervated, fibrillations will be noted. These are the spontaneous contractions of single fibers. This is the only place in the body where there is no overlying subcutaneous tissue. Hyperthyroidism and parahyperthyroidism may also cause a fibrillating tongue. If the tongue is truly atrophic its edges will be scalloped. The patient is then asked to protrude the tongue in the midline. Difficulty in protruding the tongue, deviation from the midline and involuntary movements are noted. Myotonia of the tongue can be demonstrated by having the patient place the extruded tongue on a tongue blade and then place a vertical tongue blade on the tongue which is then tapped. The indentation that occurs from the myotonic contraction may last for several seconds.

Abnormalities

Enlargement of the tongue is seen in Down's syndrome, infantile hypothyroidism, amyloid, mucopolysaccharidases and acromegaly. It is corroded after ingestion of lye or other caustic substances (not uncommon in suicide attempts). Iron deficiency anemia causes a smooth glistening tongue as do some of the autoimmune sicca syndromes (often associated with the burning tongue syndrome). Loss of the posterior circumvallate papillae with a reddened desquamative tongue is particularly prominent with B_{12} and other vitamin B deficiencies.

74

If there is unilateral denervation, longitudinal folds are prominent on the side of the muscle wasting, and the tip and median raphe curve towards the affected side when it is protruded. This is a result of the unopposed action of the contralateral genioglossus muscle. The tongue deviates to the opposite side of a supranuclear lesion (cortical or brainstem lesion). Denervation of the tongue is overwhelmingly caused by motor neuron disease. In bilateral tongue wasting, the tip and median raphe remain in the center of the mouth, it is difficult for the patient to protrude the tongue and there is gross dysarthria. Unilateral denervation of the tongue from a hypoglossal lesion causes minimal, if any, dysarthria. A small, compact-looking tongue in the floor of the mouth that is protruded with great difficulty is associated with dysarthric pseudobulbar palsy, an increased jaw jerk and spasticity which is brought about by bilateral upper motor neuron lesions.

Upper and lower motor nerve signs are combined in motor neuron disease. A trombone-like tremor on protrusion of the tongue has been noted in neurosyphilis and severe parkinsonism. Multiple abnormal tongue and mouthing movements are noted with tardive dyskinesia. Protrusion and retraction of the tongue are common with Huntington's chorea. Inability to keep the tongue protruded is more common with Sydenham's chorea.

Apraxia of tongue protrusion occurs with frontal lobe lesions as well as severe dementing illness. It may move normally during automatic speech and spontaneous licking of the lips. A short frenulum holds the tip of the tongue back which causes it to curve downward. Facial paralysis may produce a seeming deviation of the tongue to the side of the paralysis. The examiner retracts the corner of the patient's mouth to its normal position and then compares the position of the median raphe with the central incisors.

Common lesions

1 *Unilateral lower motor lesions.* Syringomyelia, poliomyelitis, isolated viral illness (Epstein–Barr virus infection, West Nile fever), schwannoma of the twelfth nerve, jugular foramen tumors, cavernous or hemangiomatous brainstem vascular malformations, trauma, high cervical enlarged lymph nodes (lymphoma); cervical fractures, motor neuron disease.
2 *Bilateral lower motor neuron lesions.* ALS, syringobulbia, rarely foramen magnum congenital defects or tumors.
3 *Bilateral upper motor neuron lesions.* Pseudobulbar palsy from bilateral brainstem vascular disease, head trauma, severe demyelinating disease acquired or metabolic (leukodystrophies), ALS.

4: The Motor System

This is perhaps the most objective component of the neurologic examination. It must be remembered that normal movement depends not only on the reflex arc of the anterior horn cell, the neuromuscular junction and muscle, but also on intact bones, joints and soft tissue. This is the foundation upon which supranuclear motor control initiates the "engram," the motor program of movement, its smoothness (cerebellum), its relation to gravity (vestibular system), the control of blood pressure in the upright position (autonomic reflexes) and the desire to move (anterior cingulate gyrus and parietal cortex). Automatic movements for walking (locomotor centers) and for emotion (amygdala, thalamus and basal ganglia) are clearly important for daily living and have an examination of their own with specific defects that point to specific pathology.

Preliminary general inspection (Figs 4.1–4.3)

The aim is to detect specific asymmetries and deformities. This is a combination of genetic defects (dysmorphism) vs acquired lesions. Trophic factors, neuritic out growth factors with guidance molecules and developmental receptors are critical. Congenital abnormalities may lead to overuse syndromes, pressure and destruction of nerve roots as they exit their spinal foramina, as well as stenosis at cervical and lumbar areas. All of the congenital defects can be diagnosed during the neurologic examination.

The patient is evaluated in the supine, sitting and erect positions. The upper extremities are placed in repose in the lap. A comparison of the size, shape and any adventitial movements are noted.

Congenital maldevelopment

Absence of muscles, asymmetry and abnormalities of muscle insertion on the limb are very important observations. The congenital neuropathies are frequently associated with high muscle insertions on the extremity that leads to thin forearms and ankles. The distal one-third of the quadriceps is atrophic, all muscles below the knee are atrophic and the leg has a "champagne bottle" appearance. In this instance, there is usually a foreshortening of the foot with reduced intrinsic foot muscles. A short neck, large or small head, kyphoscoliosis and rigid spine are associated with a very specific examination. A short neck suggests Chiari malformation (associated with a shallow posterior fossa) as well as cranial–cervical defects. A long neck with droopy shoulders (the droopy shoulder syndrome) is associated with traction on the brachial plexus. Web fingers and polydactyly (Laurence–Moon–Biedl syndrome) and a myriad of hand abnormalities from a low set thumb (Holt–Oram defect; atrioseptal defect (ASD) of the heart with possible brain abscess) to a mongolian line and trisomy 21.

Congenital absences of specific muscles (hereditary sensory motor neuron pattern (HSMN) type II, cleidocranial dysostosis) and a lower extremity with pes cavus (develops prior to age 6) suggest specific pathologies (tethered cord).

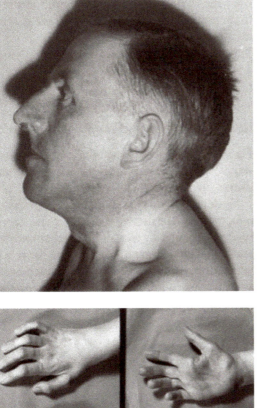

(a)

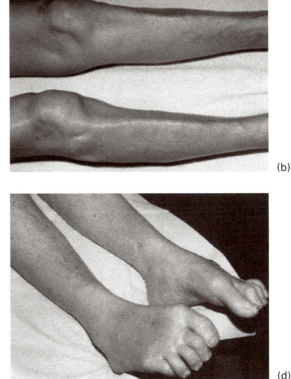

(b)

(d)

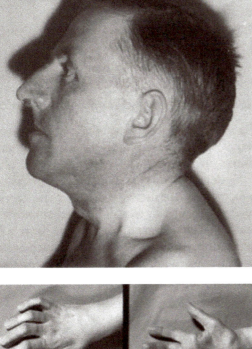

(c)

Fig. 4.1 (a) Congenital defects. Short neck. Basilar impression. Note the short retracted neck and low hairline. (b) Congenital neuropathy. Note the atrophy of the distal one-third of the quadriceps, the prominence of the tibia from atrophy of the anterior tibialis and the segmental atrophy of the gastrocnemius muscle. (c) Note the intrinsic hand muscle atrophy (dorsal and volar interossei) as well as atrophy of both thenar and hypothenar eminences. (d) Pes cavus. Note the high arch with atrophy of intrinsic foot muscle.

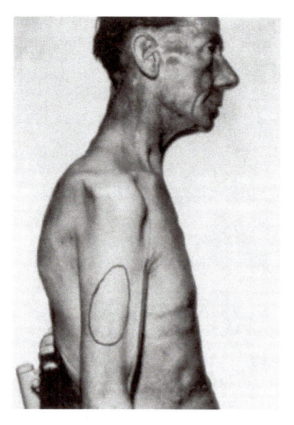

Fig. 4.2 Circumflex sensory loss, wasting of deltoid. Circumflex nerve sensory loss and periscapular wasting in neuralgic amotrophy.

Long-standing neurologic lesions

Any lower motor nerve defect in infancy causes reduced limb growth, atrophy, wasting and areflexia. An intrauterine stroke (placenta praevia) from cocaine, birth trauma or cerebral malformations cause contralateral asymmetry of development that is marked. More commonly, asymmetry is caused by neuronal migrational defects. This occurs as a result of failure of the neurons from the geminal matrix to migrate to the cerebral cortex. If the migration is halted in the white matter of the centrum semiovale, the condition is known as nodular heterotopia. There will also be nodules of neurons in the lateral ventricular wall, which are easily demonstrated by magnetic resonance imaging (MRI). If there is failure of apoptosis once the neurons have migrated to the cortex, there is a double band of neuronal tissue under the cortex (double cortex syndrome (DCS)) and failure to sculpt the cortex so it is smooth (lissencephaly *LIS I* gene) rather than gyriform. If the migration is complete but there is disorganization of the cortex at a laminar level, this is known as microdysgenesis and will not be seen on MRI. This form of symmetry is very important for diagnosis, both clinically and pathologically, of patients with complex partial seizures. Patients usually have more facial and arm smallness than leg asymmetry. They will have a poor ability to copy posture (parietal lobe function and temporal lobe spatial memory) and reflexes will be increased on the reduced growth side. Migrational defects are often syndromic and chromosomal. Asymmetry leads to kyphoscoliosis,

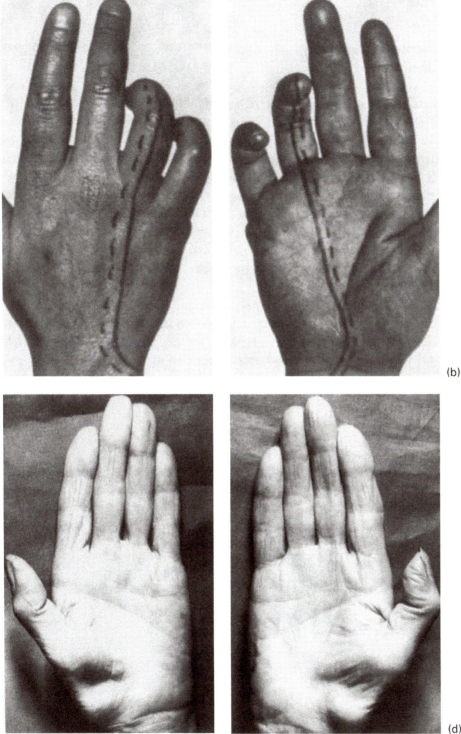

(a)

(b)

(c)

(d)

Fig. 4.3 Median/ulnar neuropathy. (a) and (b) Wasting of small muscles of hand and sensory loss resulting from ulnar nerve lesion at the elbow. Note (a) marked wasting of interossei, and (b) preservation of opponens pollicis (median nerve); (c) and (d) bilateral carpal tunnel syndrome showing typical severe wasting of both thenar eminences.

which frequently causes traction on the nerve roots that exit opposite the scoliotic curve. The combination of a disk bulge plus scoliosis may be enough to cause nerve root compression, whereas the bulge alone would not be sufficient to trap the root in the exit foramina. Severe asymmetry is associated with hemiplegia, athetoses, hyperreflexia and seizures.

Surgical lesions, particularly from modern "heavy metal" spinal fusions (pedicle screws, plates), are frequently painful at the level of the fused interspace or laterally at the offending screw level. Deformities of joints and bones with limitation of movement of the cervical and lower spine are extremely important diagnostically for all peripheral spine problems. There is a characteristic posture, spasm of muscle and weakness for each condition. It is not sufficient to note arthritis of the spine. The conditions that must be differentiated are forms of osteoarthritis and congenital defects:

1 spondylosis;
2 spinal stenosis;
3 spondylosis;
4 spondylolisthesis;
5 facet hypertrophy;
6 congenital stenosis of the cervical and lumbar spine.

All patients develop some degree of disk desiccation and bony encroachment of exit foramina with age. Unfortunately, this usually starts by the age of 40 and is severe by age 80. This normal degenerative process completely changes components of the neurologic examination. Degenerative arthritic processes of the neck are almost always associated with similar disease in the lumbosacral spine and are associated with atrophy weakness, sensory loss, ataxia and reflex changes.

Examination of joint movement

This part of the examination is neglected by all except rheumatologists and orthopedic physicians. Charcot's joints (completely denervated and often painless) are rarely seen from tertiary syphilis in the modern age. They are more commonly seen as a manifestation of a cervical syrinx, diabetes or amyloid neuropathy. Severe ulnar deviation of the hands with distinctive small joint lesions will invariably be accompanied by intrinsic hand muscle weakness and atrophy as well as the possibility of spondylolisthesis of C2–C3 or pannus formation at this level (destroys the cruciate ligament).

Examination of spinal movement to all planes is dramatically important in the evaluation of any patient with back and leg pain. The examiner notes the degree of flexion, extension or lateral mobility that is lost. No patient with lumbar stenosis flexes well. No patient with congenital or acquired cervical stenosis has normal lateral movement or extension of the neck. In a patient with lumbar spondylolisthesis, there is a characteristic pelvic tilt and pain both with straight leg raising and with extension. Stance, posture and the spinal examination are discussed in detail later.

Local inspection of muscle (Fig. 4.4)

Inspection of the shoulder, hip, forearm, legs and calf muscles allows the examiner to decide if the patient has:

1. proximal or distal myopathy;
2. anterior horn cell disease;
3. a symmetrical motor neuropathy;
4. focal nerve disease or a radiculopathy.

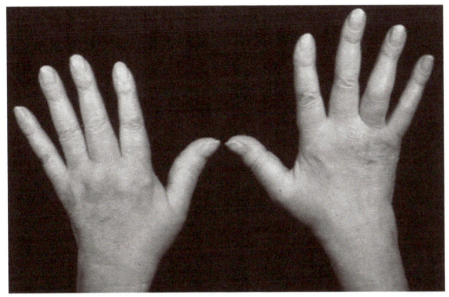

(ai)

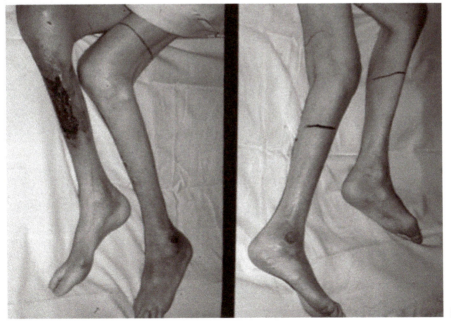

(aii)

Fig. 4.4 (ai) Early anterior horn cell disease with wasting of the first dorsal interosseous muscle. (aii) Wasting resulting from severe peripheral neuropathy. All muscles below the knee are wasted but the distal one-third of the quadriceps is normal. Neurogenic ulcers are present. (*Cont'd on page 82*).

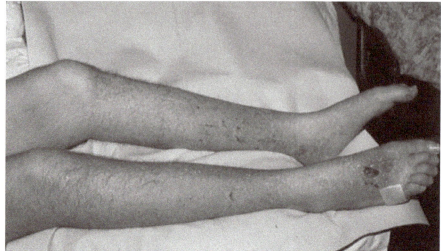

(aiii)

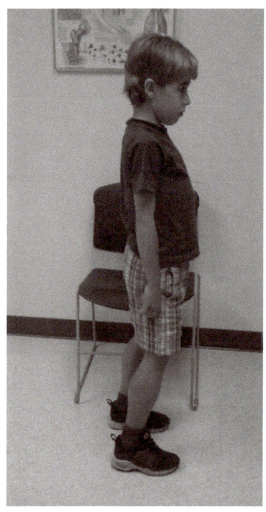

(b)

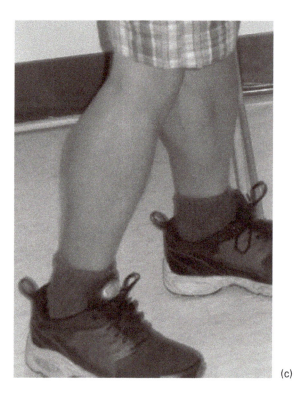

(c)

Fig. 4.4 (*cont'd*) (aiii) Rocker bottom boot of congenital neuropathy. Note the distal one-third of the quadriceps muscle neurogenic ulcer and flat foot. (b) Note the lordotic curve and associated protuberant abdomen. (c) Enlarged pseudohypertrophic calves.

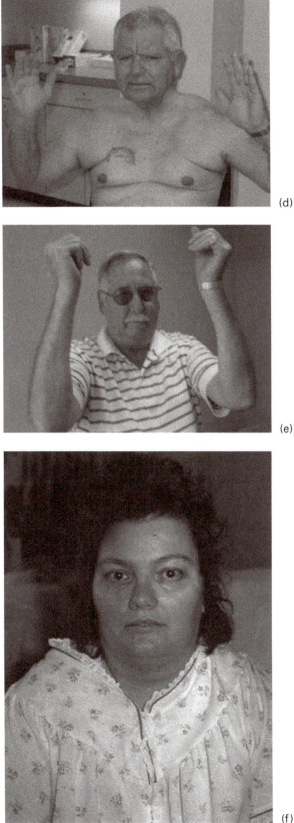

Fig. 4.4 (*cont'd*) (d) Note the transverse smile, prominent weakness and atrophy of biceps and triceps with relative spacing of the deltoids. Axillary areas are proximal because of pectoral muscle atrophy. (e) Inclusion body myopathy. Note atrophy of the form flexor muscles with flexion contraction of the fingers. (f) Note the molar rash and capillary inflammation around the eyes.

Proximal weakness is characteristic of acquired and hereditary myopathy, fasciculations, motor neuron disease, first dorsal interosseous wasting, ulnar neuropathy, symmetrical wasting of small muscles of the hands and feet, common medical issues such as rheumatoid arthritis and diabetes mellitus. Rarely, there is muscle hypertrophy in adults. These illnesses include the dystrophinopathies, hypothyroidism (Hoffmann's syndrome), hyperkalemic periodic paralysis, congenital myotonias or Isaac's syndrome. Unilateral hypertrophy has rarely been described with neuropathic processes (Kugelberg–Welander neuropathy and radiculopathy). Wasting is noted by comparison side to side of individual muscles and by the examiner's evaluation of what is normally expected for the age, occupation and size of the patient. The eminences of the hand are important. Carpal tunnel syndrome, with median nerve compression, destroys the abductor pollicis brevis, whereas rheumatoid arthritis and navicular bone arthritis also affect the opponens and adductor muscles. A scooped or extremely wasted thenar eminence suggests severe C8 radiculopathy. Hypothenar eminence wasting occurs with ulnar nerve neuropathy and destruction of thoracic 1 (T1).

Wasting occurs with axonal and anterior horn cell disease rather than by compression or demyelination of nerves. In the former, it is associated with fasciculation. In the lower extremity, the anterior tibialis muscle should be rounded adjacent to the tibia. Gentle pressure of the tibia demonstrates wasting. The gastrocnemius muscle should be convex when the leg is raised from the bed. It frequently appears normal if the leg is only examined resting on the bed. The extensor digitorum brevis of the lateral foot is an excellent muscle to evaluate for S1 root disease. The examiner should note the prominence of tendons and the arch of the foot, pes cavus being prominent with congenital neuropathy. Approximately 10% of patients with congenital neuropathy have no arch ("rocker bottom" foot). Wasting of the caps of the shoulder (deltoid) is physiologic in elderly patients as cervical spondylosis frequently affects C4–C5 and C5–C6 roots. Atrophy of the supraspinatus and infraspinatus muscles, normal in elderly patients, causes prominence of the scapula and spine.

Types of muscle wasting

Generalized wasting

Generalized systemic illness such as congestive heart failure, liver and renal failure as well as malignancy are associated with type II muscle atrophy and have a proximal predominance. The muscles may be much stronger than their appearances. Critical care myopathy affects proximal muscles and the diaphragm. It is always a possibility in those patients who are difficult to wean from respirators. It is often associated with axonal critical care neuropathy which causes generalized wasting.

Amyotrophic lateral sclerosis (ALS) causes severe wasting in its later stages. It is associated with fasciculations and wasting of the tongue, hyperactive reflexes and Babinski's responses. End stage myopathy of all types, with the exception of many of the congenital myopathies, is associated with wasting. Mitochondrial muscle disease is associated more with fatigue while metabolic muscle disease causes cramping rather than wasting. Prolonged exercise that induces cramps is most suggestive of muscle disease associated with faculty beta oxidation of fat. There is no muscle wasting.

Proximal muscle wasting

Wasting occurs in muscles that are weak in the inflammatory myopathies. Occasionally, distal muscles are affected in primary acquired inflammatory myopathy. Atrophy of the anterior tibialis and brachioradialis (act as if they were proximal muscles) muscle atrophy may occur with the polymyositis/dermatomyositis complex.

Facial, ocular and neck muscle involvement occur with:

1 congenital myopathies such as nemaline, myotubular and centronuclear myopathy;

2 myotonic dystrophy, oculopharyngeal dystrophy and fascioscapulohumeral dystrophy;

3 mitochondrial myopathies such as Kearns–Sayre and myoclonic epilepsy with ragged red fibers (MERFF).

Distal muscle wasting occurs on a congenital basis with Welander's, Miyoshi and Nonaka dystrophy, as well as myopathy with inclusion bodies.

Duchenne and Becker muscular dystrophies

All dystrophinopathies result from mutations of the dystrophin gene on the short arm of the X chromosome. The protein dystrophin is the product of the gene and is part of a larger associated glycoprotein complex which is called the dystrophin-associated protein complex (DAP). DAP and dystrophin connect the intracellular cytoskeletal protein actin to the basal laminae through the extracellular matrix. This complex is believed to stabilize the sarcolemmal membrane during contraction. The DAP complex is composed of a dystroglycan, sarcoglycan and syntropic group. Most Duchenne and Becker muscular dystrophy mutations are deletions.

In Duchenne muscular dystrophy (DMD), boys are usually noted to be weak at 2–3 years of age with primary difficulty with walking. They demonstrate a waddling gait at 3–6 years of age, and have difficulty with running, jumping and climbing stairs. Lumbar lordosis and calf hypertrophy are common. The calf muscles have an unusual rubbery consistency to them. Gower's maneuver is common (patients use their hands to push up from the thighs) (Fig. 4.5). Neck flexor weakness is present at all stages of the illness. A child with DMD cannot lift the head against gravity, which

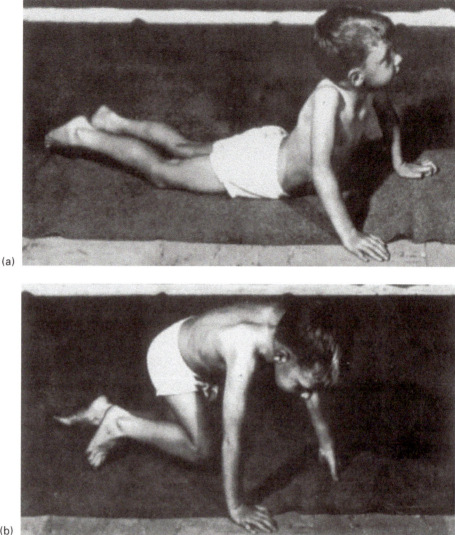

(a)

(b)

Fig. 4.5 Gower's maneuver. Gower's sign, the characteristic method of rising from the floor.

distinguishes it from Becker muscular dystrophy (BMD) and outliers. Pseudohypertrophy can be seen in gluteal, deltoid and masseter muscles as well as the calves. Early in the disease the process is true hypertrophy, but over time muscles are replaced by fat and connective tissue which gives them their rubbery consistency. Plantar flexors and inverters remain strong over the course of the disease while the anterior tibialis muscle weakens. Heel cord contractures result. Muscle strength decreases between 6 and 11 years and reflexes are hard to elicit in the following pattern: triceps > biceps > knees > brachioradialis and ankle. Joint contractures, cardiac and pulmonary diseases supervene and the patient is wheelchair-bound by age 12. Cranial and sphincter muscles are spared while heart muscle, brain and smooth muscle are affected.

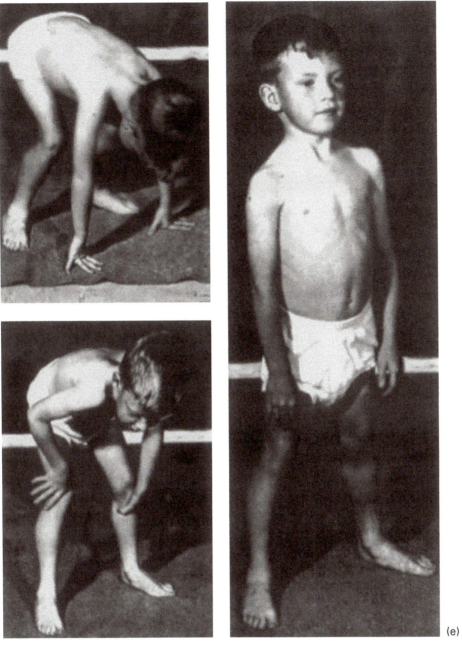

(c)

(d)

(e)

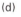

Fig. 4.5 (*cont'd*)

BMD demonstrates a later onset of symptoms with a similar muscular pattern of weakness. Pelvic and thigh muscles are involved first although calf hypertrophy is also seen. There is less weakness of tibialis anterior and peroneal muscles. There is relative preservation of neck flexor strength; contractures and scoliosis are less common as is cardiac and cognitive dysfunction. Cardiac disease can present prior to skeletal weakness. These patients survive to adulthood and are ambulatory beyond 16 years of age. Death occurs usually between 30 and 60 years of age from cardiomyopathy or respiratory insufficiency.

Emery–Dreifuss muscular dystrophy

This dystrophy is inherited as an X-linked (EMD1) and an autosomal dominant (AD) (EMD2) form that encodes emerin in which there is a mutation in the lamina A/C gene. There are three major presentations:
1 muscle weakness;
2 contractures;
3 cardiac onset with sudden death.

Muscle wasting is often most severe in a humeroperoneal distribution. Some patients have hypertrophy of the extensor digitorum brevis muscle concomitant with prominent posterior leg wasting. There may be selective weakness of elbow flexion and finger extension. The muscle wasting may be most prominent in the posterior compartment of the leg and contractures of the quadratus lumborum of the lower back cause a rigid spine. Adult patients have flexion contractions of the wrist, elbows, ankles and neck. Cardiac involvement occurs between the second to fourth decades (EMD1) and third to fourth decades in (EMD2). The major features are atrial paralysis and dilated cardiomyopathy.

Fasicoscapular muscular dystrophy

Fasicoscapular muscular dystrophy (FSMD) has now been mapped to chromosome 4q 35 and is secondary to deletion of a repetitive element which are known as D4Z4 repeats.

The disease is clinically evident in the second decade of life, although up to 30% of patients may be asymptomatic. The usual pattern of weakness is that of concomitant scapula fixator and facial weakness. Patients cannot whistle, sip through a straw or blow out their cheeks. Their eyes are slightly open when they sleep. There is a descending rostral caudal weakness, facial, shoulder girdle, peroneal and hip girdle. Patients have wide palpebral fissures, poor facial expression and a transverse smile. Neck flexor muscles are relatively spared compared to extensors. The shoulders are forward sloped and rounded with pectoral atrophy and axillary creases. The scapulae are winged and laterally displaced with preferential wasting of the lower trapezius muscles. The biceps and triceps are wasted out of proportion to the deltoids ("Popeye" appearance). There is preferential weakness of lower abdominal muscles causing upward deviation of the umbilicus with neck flexion (Beevor's sign) (Fig. 4.6). This is specific for FSMD in muscle disease. Foot dorsiflexion is involved with gastrocnemius sparing. Reflexes are depressed. Hearing loss and retinal telangiectasia are associated. Approximately 5% of patients have cardiac involvement with conduction defects. The abnormalities are primarily supraventricular tachyarrhythmias.

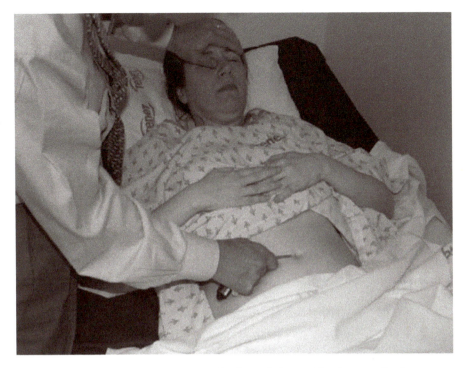

Fig. 4.6 Beevor's sign. The examiner marks the umbilicus with a key or reflex hammer. The patient then flexes the neck against resistance. The umbilicus is at a dermatomal level of T10. If the umbilicus moves up the rectus, abdominal muscles at T11 and T12 are weak. If the umbilicus moves downward, the rectus abdominal muscles at T8 and T9 are weak. The umbilicus moves approximately 1 cm under these circumstances.

Early anterior tibialis and hip muscle weakness with subtle facial weakness can make the diagnosis difficult. The usual misdiagnoses are scapuloperoneal syndromes or limb girdle dystrophies.

Distinctive features to be sought are:
1 asymmetry of weakness;
2 sparing of deltoids;
3 relative sparing of neck flexors;
4 straight clavicles;
5 Beevor's sign (lower abdominal weakness);
6 high-frequency hearing loss or retinal vasculopathy.

Scapuloperoneal syndromes

This is descriptive designation of a heterogeneous group of disorders that may be either neurogenic or myogenic in etiology. It is likely that some patients with a scapuloperoneal phenotype are variants of FSMD.

Limb girdle muscular dystrophy

There is no absolute clinical or scientific consensus of what constitutes a limb girdle myopathy. Molecular genetic diagnosis will determine this classification in the future. A guide that may be useful for the present is the onset of weakness in the pelvic or shoulder girdle or both concomitantly. Early contractures may be seen in some AD inherited forms, but rarely with autosomal recessive (AR) disease. Calf hypertrophy is common, but shows intrafamilial variability. Exclusion criteria are onset in distal, facial or extraocular muscles although they may be affected as the illness progresses. Onset of weakness occurs at any age. In AR kindreds, the onset is in the early twenties. Later onset occurs in AD disease. In general, limb girdle muscular dystrophies are slowly progressive. Many patients have a normal life span although some die before middle age. AD patients, in general, have a slower course.

The sarcoglycan (SG) and dystroglycan subunits (DG) are membrane glycoproteins that are synthesized in the endoplasmic reticulum. The four SG subunits form the SG complex. The sarcoglycanopathies are caused by mutations of sarcoglycan genes. If one gene is mutated there is a reduction of all SG subunits. The diseases associated with SG gene mutations are termed limb girdle muscular dystrophies (LGMD 2C–2F). The sarcoglycans may have a functional role in signal transduction. The diseases associated with each loss of a sarcoglycan subunit are:

1 LGMD 2D – α sarcoglycan;
2 LGMD 2E – β sarcoglycan;
3 LGMD 2C – sarcoglycanopathy;
4 LGMD 2F;
5 δ-sarcoglycanopathy.

Calpainopathy – LGMD 2A

The disease was first described from the Reunion Islands of the West Indian Ocean. The gene is calpain-3 (chromosome 15q2–21.1), which expresses a non-lysosomal calcium-dependent proteinase. It is now known to occur in a worldwide distribution. The age of onset is 3–30 years of age with a mean of 10 years. The early stages manifest gluteus maximus and thigh adductor weakness. The quadriceps is minimally involved. Abdominal muscles are more affected than spinal muscles with consequent lordosis. There is rare hypertrophy of the calves. Weakness and atrophy of periscapular muscles supervene and contractures develop in the elbows, hips and knees.

Dysferlinopathy – LGMD 2B

This AR LGMD has been mapped to chromosome 2p. Miyoshi distal myopathy has been mapped to 2p12–p14. Large kindreds with myopathy mapped to 2p demonstrated that some members have Miyoshi distal myopathy and some had proximal LGMD 2B. The age of onset ranged from 13 to 35 years of age. Upper extremity weakness follows that noted in proximal muscles of the lower extremities.

The AD LGMDs are quite similar in presentation to the AR diseases. The genetic evaluation directs the examiner to which category of limb girdle dystrophy is present. Distinctive features are the contractures of Bethlehem myopathy and LGMD 4C which are distinguished from Emery–Dreifuss muscular dystrophy by the absences of heart block.

Proximal muscle wasting can be a feature of Kugelberg–Welander disease (an anterior horn cell illness), severe inflammatory polymyositis/dermatomyositis (PM/DM) complex as well as selected metabolic, congenital and mitochondrial myopathies.

Motor neuron disease occasionally affects the shoulder girdle with fasciculations, wasting and weakness prior to its expression in distal muscles. Syringomyelia of the cervical spine is associated with a dissociated sensory loss, pain and temperature defects greater than touch, segmental wasting with absent reflexes of the upper extremities and increased reflexes in the knees and ankles. Neuralgia amyotrophica, probably a viral or autoimmune process, asymmetrically wastes an upper extremity. It may be bilateral and progress for months. Preceding events include vaccination, injury or a viral illness. It often is extremely painful. There may be sensory loss in the axillary nerve distribution of the affected side. Rarely, the diaphragm is affected.

Proximal muscle weakness and wasting in practice is most often the polymyositis/dermatomyositis complex or that associated with collagen vascular diseases such as systemic lupus erythematosus (SLE). In dermatomyositis, the rash is over the extensor surfaces of the joints of the hand. Periungual telangiectasia is typical of SLE while features of scleroderma and SLE occur with mixed collagen vascular disease. Muscles are usually not tender with inflammatory myopathies. Swallowing is often affected in the PM/DM complex.

Compressive lesions of the cervical cord occur most commonly at C5–C6 more than C4–C5 and may be associated with deltoid and spinatus atrophy, loss of biceps reflexes with exaggerated triceps or finger flexion reflexes. There is invariant decreased neck movement, it is held in a forward flexed posture and there is usually some slight sensory loss.

Cauda equina lesions are most often caused by disk extrusion, neoplasms and now cytomegalovirus (CMV) infection in patients with HIV. They may cause wasting of gluteal muscles, perineal sensory loss and sphincter incontinence.

Distal muscle wasting

Almost all of the conditions that cause proximal wasting in later stages cause distal wasting. Distal wasting occurs primarily with anterior horn cell disease, motor axon diseases and a group of distal myopathies. The examiner needs to carefully examine the tongue for atrophy and fibrillation, inspect the muscles for fasciculations at rest, percuss them to induce fasciculations if they are hyperexcitable and check carefully for sensory loss.

Distal wasting of the forearm and intrinsic hand muscles

Wasting of the intrinsic hand muscles results from lesions anywhere from the anterior horn cells of C8–T1 (C8 for the thenar eminence and T1 for the hypothenar eminence) to the site of innervation of the muscles. Anterior horn cell involvement at cervical levels is most often a result of motor neuron disease, syringomyelia, cervical cord tumors and, rarely, poliomyelitis or West Nile fever. The ventral roots at these cervical segments are compromised by cervical spondylosis (osteophytes in the exit foramina; more common at C5–C6 levels), cervical tumors and now described with abiotrophies (failure to sustain anterior horn cell survival by lack of trophic factors or survival genes) and demyelinating disease. The inflammation of white matter tracts may directly affect anterior horn cells or they may die because of peripheral loss of their axons. Brachial plexus trauma from vehicular accidents, neurologic amyotrophy or autoimmune destruction may damage C8–T1 with consequent intrinsic hand muscle atrophy. In the rib-band syndrome of Gilliat, a fibrous band compresses T1 in the thoracic outlet. Sulcal tumors particularly from carcinoma of the lung or breast catch the lower trunk of the plexus at the apex of the lung. A Horner's syndrome is frequently noted. Traumatic compression of the median, ulnar and radial nerves at different levels affects specific intrinsic hand and forearm muscles.

Autoimmune neuropathies, particularly those secondary to ganglioside M1 (GM1) and monoclonal antibody glycoprotein (MAG) antibodies, may affect the upper extremities prior to the lower extremities. Acute intermittent porphyria frequently causes severe wasting of forearm and intrinsic hand muscles which rapidly returns to normal at the end of an attack.

Median nerve compression at the carpal tunnel causes wasting of the thenar eminence (primarily the abductor pollicis brevis). The sensory loss is most severe at the tip of the index finger. Damage to the ulnar nerve at the cubital tunnel (elbow) causes severe wasting of intrinsic hand muscles with the exception of the opponens pollicis and abductor pollicis brevis which are innervated by the median nerve. The sensory loss splits the fourth finger. If there is compression at Guyon's canal at the wrist (entrance of the ulnar nerve to the hand) there may be no wasting or sensory loss, but a positive Tinel's sign (mechanical hypersensitivity to tapping) may reproduce the symptom. The nerve at this level may be compressed by a spur of the piriform bone, trauma or a ganglion cyst.

The genes for the AD distal myopathies are rapidly being identified. They include AD late onset forms of Welander's (2p13) with initial weakness of the hands, finger and wrist and the AD Marksberry/Griggs/Udd variant (2q13) with early involvement of the anterior leg compartment. The AR Nonaka myopathy localized to chromosome 9p1 also affects the anterior lower leg compartment. AR or sporadic Miyoshi distal myopathy affects the posterior compartment of the leg. Miyoshi and variants may have early adult onsets. Distal myopathy with vocal cord paralysis and pharyngeal weakness has its onset in the fourth to sixth decades, is AD and has been mapped to chromosome 5q3. The anterior compartment of the legs and finger extensors are involved first. Myofibular myopathy is undergoing a reclassification and may start in either the hands or legs.

The most common primarily distal myopathy is myotonic dystrophy. This is easily distinguished by the characteristic "hang jaw" and facial features, frontal balding, stellate cataracts, cognitive difficulties, cardiac abnormalities and myotonia.

Other myopathies with distal weakness include:

1 FSMD;

2 scapuloperoneal syndromes;

3 congenital myopathies (nemaline, central core, centronuclear); metabolic myopathies (debrancher deficiency and acid maltase deficiency); oculopharyngeal and Emery–Dreifuss muscular dystrophy.

In polymyositis, the usual wasting and weakness is proximal. However, the brachioradialis and anterior tibialis muscles may be involved. The second most common inflammatory myopathy in elderly patients is inclusion body myopathy which is characterized by forearm wasting and intrinsic hand muscle wasting with finger flexor contractures.

The lower leg

The distal myopathies strike the anterior or posterior compartments of the lower leg. Characteristically, the hereditary motor sensory neuropathies and the Charcot–Marie–Tooth subcategories of these entities have characteristic pes cavus (90%) or "rocker bottom" feet (10%). In general, the distal one-third of the quadriceps is atrophic and all muscles below the knee are affected. L4–L5 radiculopathy causes wasting of the anterior tibialis muscle. This is easily seen as a depression next to the tibia. S1 radiculopathy wastes the gastrocnemius muscle (medial side more prominently).

Peripheral wasting of both upper and lower extremities (Fig. 4.7)

Chronic metabolic or distal "dying back" neuropathies from diabetes, renal, liver, thyroid or toxic causes all result in rather symmetric distal atrophy, sensory loss, autonomic dysregulation and reflex loss. These are distinguished from the HSMNs by family history, foot abnormalities, kyphoscoliosis and the other neurologic signs associated with each form of neuropathy. Diabetes has a penchant for first dorsal interosseous atrophy (probable subclinical ulnar neuropathy) in association with generalized loss of reflexes of muscles that may not be clinically weak.

Muscle tone

The patient needs to be relaxed. The examiner flexes and extends the fingers and wrists while talking to the patient. If basal ganglia disease is suspected, the examiner rotates the wrist while asking the patient to open

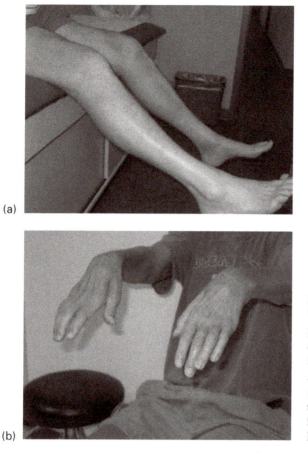

(a)

(b)

Fig. 4.7 (a) Distal myopathy. Welander's variant. Note the prominence of foot tendons and early atrophy of all muscles below the knee. (b) Amyotrophic lateral sclerosis (ALS). Note the prominent scalloping of the first dorsal interossei and all intrinsic hand muscles.

and close the opposite hand (reinforcement). This will cause a cog or interruption of tone in the examined extremity ("cog-wheel" rigidity). If it is equally difficult to extend and flex the arm against resistance the patient has ("lead-pipe") rigidity. The clasp knife phenomenon is extremely difficult to demonstrate. The patient may have an increase of tone on extension of the arm that suddenly breaks because of 1b fiber inhibition from tendons that project to inhibitory interneurons or the anterior horn cells themselves and the tone suddenly lessens. Shaking the hands gently as if you are drying them often demonstrates hypotonicity. In an unconscious patient, dropping a raised arm and evaluating the speed of its fall is helpful in evaluating symmetries of tone.

Testing tone in the lower limb

First roll the limbs with the palm of the hands on the skin. This evaluates the tone of the hip girdle musculature. During the maneuver evaluate the side-to-side movement of the feet. Excess movement indicates reduced tone. Pick the leg up and shake it gently while observing the feet. This is a similar method and often times more effective. If the patient is in bed, place the hands in the popliteal fossa and quickly raise the knee. As the knee is raised, the foot should slide up the bed, if it is raised off the bed there is increased tone. Observe the manner in which the leg slides back towards its original position. If there is a delay, tone is increased ("Queen Square sign").

Loss of tone

The muscles are lax, there is decreased resistance to passive movement; the limb is displaced too easily and does not check with sudden release. The tendon reflexes are often decreased (there are notable exceptions). Loss of tone occurs by breaking the reflex arc (no input to anterior horn cells) or the firing from anterior horn cells is decreased which occurs with cerebellar disease, spinal or cerebral shock (decrease of facilitation of anterior horn cells which decreases the drive of the gamma loop). The gamma loop controls the muscle spindle. When activated, the intrafusal fibers of the spindle contract which in turn brings the anterior horn cell closer to depolarization and discharges some with consequent muscle contraction. Not enough muscles fire to move the joint, but muscle tone is increased.

Common causes of hypotonia

1 *Lesions of the motor side of the reflex arc.* Examples are pure lower motor neuron disease such as poliomyelitis, West Nile virus and primary spino-muscular atrophy. In ALS, the upper motor neurons are involved and there is disinhibition of the gamma loop which increases reflexes and tone. Motor neuropathy that occurs with GM1 and MAG antibodies to epitopes on muscle axons as well as acute motor axonopathy (AMAN), Guillain–Barré syndrome (GBS) and peripheral nerve injury all decrease tone.

2 *Lesions of the sensory side of the reflex arc.* Sensory neuropathies, tabes dorsalis, small fiber neuropathies that include those from antisulfatide epitopes, anti-Hu antibodies in response to a tumor antigen (paraneoplastic), amyloid (TTR met 30-transthyretin), pyridoxine and other toxins decrease tone. Large fiber neuropathies decrease tone more than small fiber ones.

3 *Combined motor and sensory lesions.* Syringomyelia, cord or root lesions, or any cause of spinal or cerebral shock, such as large internal capsule strokes or hemorrhage, all decrease tone.

4 *Lesion of the muscle itself.* This can be caused by many of the myopathies: acquired, mitochondrial and dystrophic. The dystrophies frequently affect the intrafusal fibers that control the muscle spindle (the more lax the intrafusal fiber the harder it is to fire the anterior horn cell that contracts the muscle). This phenomenon is especially true in DMD, BMD, FSMD and oculopharyngeal dystrophy. In hypokalemic periodic paralysis, the patient is paralyzed and areflexic, but the muscles feel tense and swollen (because of water in the T-tubule system).

5 *Cerebellar lesions.* Hypotonia is common and is accompanied by pendular reflexes and hypometric pursuit eye movements (the eye seems to lag the object as it is moved through the visual field). The hypometria is not marked. Failure to check (resist) displacement of the extremities is always present.

6 *Chorea.* Sydenham's and Huntington's chorea patients also are hypotonic. The collagen disorders of Marfan's disease, homocystinuria, osteogenic imperfecta, Ehlers–Danlos type IV are associated with hyperextensibility of distal extremity joints and hypotonia.

Increase of tone

1 *Spasticity.* In this condition, tone and resistance of muscle lengthening in one group of muscles are greater than another. Rarely, a "clasp knife" phenomenon occurs in which the movement against resistance suddenly decreases (because of activation of 1b afferents to the anterior horn cell). Spasticity most frequently occurs in the lower extremities and is associated with hyperactive and reduplicative reflexes (clonus) as well as Babinski's sign. In the upper extremity, a "supinator catch" may be demonstrated by supination and pronation of the forearm. Spastic muscles are frequently contracted at rest, are firm and cause contractures. An increase of adductor tone in spastic paraparesis causes a characteristic scissors gait.

2 *Lead pipe or plastic rigidity.* This is caused by equal resistance of agonist and antagonist muscles. In many akinetic rigid dementing illnesses, limbs are almost fixed and it is difficult to extend or flex the extremities. This state is often accompanied by a forward flexed posture and release of degenerative cortical reflexes. The gait is hesitant and cautious as the swing phase is shortened (Wells' dementia gait). There is often associated apraxia of gait and a "magnetic" foot grasp (normal pressure hydrocephalus).

3 *"Cog-wheel" rigidity.* This is caused by alternate contraction of agonists and antagonists. A catch to the movement is noted (Negri's sign). It is most easily noted at the wrist which is rotated. Opening and closing the opposite hand ("reinforcement") often accentuates or brings out the sign. It is often most noticeable at the onset of the induced movements and is extremely helpful in early Parkinson's disease.

Clonus

Sudden stretching of a disinhibited muscle induces repetitive reflex contractions which are often caused by a supranuclear lesion of the pyramidal tract. It may be evident in any muscle, but is most easily seen in the legs. The ankle is suddenly or rhythmically extended, which induces the repetitive contractures. It may be easily seen in the quadriceps muscle by displacing the patella sharply downward. Extremely nervous patients may demonstrate the sign. It is associated with weakness, poor fractionated movement and hyperactive reflexes. Spasticity and Babinski's or Hoffman's signs are often associated.

Lesions producing increased tone

A lesion of the corticospinal system (or upper motor neuron) whether at its origin or in the spinal cord produces spasticity, increased tendon reflexes, a loss of abdominal reflexes and Babinski's sign. Spasticity is most often seen following anoxic birth injury, vascular disease of a hemisphere, tumors, degenerative disease, demyelinating and autoimmune disease of myelin or neurologic conditions in which myelin was not formed properly (phenylketonuria). It frequently follows injuries to the brain or spinal cord. The gamma system that controls tone is disinhibited.

In general, these findings hold true in clinical practice. The cortex is biased toward inhibition (there are 10 times the number of inhibitory GABAergic interneurons that synapse on descending corticospinal neurons than excitatory glutamatergic neurons). A mammalian system is a spring ready for rapid release, the opposite of a reptile which has to warm up with the sun in order to move. A primary cortical lesion may cause instant hyperactive reflexes because of the greater loss of GABAergic inhibition on projecting neurons. The deeper into the brain a lesion occurs (basal ganglia hemorrhage) the more likely the patient is to suffer "brain shock" with loss of descending excitation to anterior horn cells and consequent decreased tone.

Lead pipe or plastic rigidity (increased tone of agonists and antagonists) occurs with all forms of akinetic parkinsonian syndromes. These include striatonigral degeneration, multiple system atrophy, progressive supranuclear palsy (the head is extended rather than flexed to utilize the vestibular ocular reflexes to move the eyes down as the patient cannot voluntarily do so) and corticobasal ganglia degeneration. In the past, it was common with reserpine and chlorpromazine usage as well as carbon monoxide poisoning. It occurs rarely with basal ganglia neoplasms and catatonia. Cog-wheel rigidity also occurs in all forms of parkinsonian syndromes but is most helpful in Parkinson's disease in the early stages.

Extrapyramidal rigidity in a slight form is a concomitant of aging. Joint and muscle contractures can give the impression of increased tone. Patients with loss of postural and proprioception that occurs abruptly seek support when being examined and give the false impression of having increased tone. The examiner is passively trying to move the extremity and the patient appears to be pushing against them. This may also be a problem with the subjective visual vertical (SVV). This refers to the patients' own sense of where they are in regard to the vertical plane. If the patient feels this is off, usually slowly learning toward the examiner, he or she will try to right themself to the midline and push against the examiner (a "pusher").

Myotonia

Myotonia is continued muscle contraction following a specific movement. The patient with facial myotonia cannot open the eyes following a cough nor rapidly open the hand after clenching the fist. It can be elicited by percussion of an involved muscle. It is striking when the index or long finger remain extended following percussion of the extensor profundus muscles of the forearm. Percussion of the thenar eminence causes adduction of the thumb and persistent dimpling of the muscle. The myoedema phenomenon occurs with hypothyroidism, marasmus hypokalemia and low albumin states. Hard percussion of a myotonic muscle causes dimpling followed by a raised lump on the side of the dimple.

Myotonic states: myotonic dystrophy

The myotonias are categorized as those with dystrophic features and those without. The classic myotonic dystrophy is associated with frontal baldness, wasting of masseter temporalis and pterygoid muscles that produce the characteristic "hang dog" or "hatchet jaw" facies, as well as atrophy of distal extremity sternocleidomastoid muscles. Cataracts, a flat glucose tolerance curve, small testicles, high follicle-stimulating hormone (FSH) levels and cognitive impairment complete the clinical picture. Recently, a proximal form of the disease with fewer systemic features (DM2) has been described.

The Schwartz–Jampel syndrome is an AR, sex-linked dystrophic form of the illness with short stature and contractures. The underlying defect in these illnesses is a chloride channel abnormality that causes repetitive firing of the sarcolemmal membrane.

The congenital myotonias are characterized by hypertrophied muscles with myotonia also affecting cranial muscles. They have no dystrophic features. Thomsen's disease is AD while Becker's is AR and tends to be less severe. There are several sodium (Na) channel myotonias that fluctuate and are potassium sensitive. These also are without dystrophic features. Myotonia is a feature of paramyotonia congenita and hyperkalemic periodic paralysis. Paramyotonia congenita patients demonstrate dramatic myotonia on exposure to cold which also is a feature of hyperkalemic periodic paralysis, but to a lesser degree.

Muscle power

Muscle testing requires placing the muscle in a position in which its primary action can be evaluated. The grading of muscle power is usually denoted on a 0–5 scale, with a 5/5 muscle as completely normal. A 0/5 muscle is paralyzed; 1/5 denotes a flicker of movement; 2/5 is a muscle that can move slightly on the bed; 3/5 is a muscle that can just sustain itself against gravity; 4/5 is a slightly weak muscle.

The patient is asked to make the specific movement required to demonstrate the action of that muscle and to maintain it against the full effort of the examiner to overcome it. The questions that are answered by the examination are as follow:

1 Is the muscle as strong as expected for its size and the body habitus of the patient?

2 Is it different from its contralateral counterpart?

3 What is its degree of weakness, if any?

4 Is the weakness constant or variable?

5 Does it improve with rest?

The bias of many examiners is that patients are hysterical and feigning symptoms and signs. In my experience, this is rare and when it occurs it is easy to diagnose. The question should be whether this patient is weak and it is the job of the examiner to demonstrate the specific muscle weakness.

Routine tests of muscle groups

The examination of major muscle groups includes the flexors and extensors of the neck; the adductors, abductors and rotators of the shoulder; the flexors and extensors of the elbow, wrist and fingers; abdominal muscles and extensors of the spine; the flexors and extensors of the hip and knee; the dorsiflexors and plantar flexors of the feet; and the flexors and extensors of the toes.

This examination starts with an evaluation of the patient leaving the chair that he or she was sitting in during the history taking and walking into the examining room. Difficulty getting out of the chair suggests proximal myopathy. An abnormality of gait will quickly help to localize a major underlying pathologic process such as hemiplegia, basal ganglia dysfunction, a spastic process or the peripheral weakness of a steppage gait. The patient changes and then is asked to walk on heels (anterior tibialis and extensors of the foot), on the toes (gastrocnemius and soleus), the major flexors of the foot and to get out of a squat which engages the gluteus maximus. Thus, within 15–30 seconds, the examiner has evaluated most of the lower extremity. If weakness is noted in any muscle group, the examiner tests each individual muscle of that group to determine the pattern of weakness. Is this primarily a peripheral process such as a proximal myopathy or a distal neuropathy, a lesion of the root, plexus or nerve or a lesion of the CNS? The individual muscle weakness demonstrated has to be placed into the context of associated findings which include:

1 fasciculation or atrophy;

2 sensory loss;

3 tone;

4 reflex abnormality.

Muscles of the head and neck

The method of examination of the facial muscles, the masseters, temporalis and sternocleidomastoids and trapezius are described under the cranial nerve examination. The neck flexors and extensors are very helpful in detecting muscle, neuromuscular junction and anterior horn cell disease. Most primary myopathies affect flexors of the neck to a greater degree than extensors, which is the reverse of anterior horn cell disease. Extensor weakness maybe so marked in this instance that the patient is unable to raise the head from the chest ("dropped head syndrome"). Neuromuscular disease, primarily myasthenia gravis, may affect both flexors and extensors of the neck to a similar degree.

Testing of muscles of the shoulder girdle and scapula through muscles of the great toe are demonstrated in Figs 4.7–4.50.

Muscles of the shoulder girdle and scapula

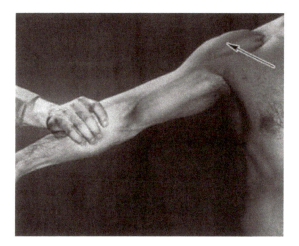

Fig. 4.8 Muscle: deltoid. Main segmental nerve supply: C5. Peripheral nerve: circumflex or axillary nerve. Test: the patient holds the arm abducted to 60° against the examiner's resistance.

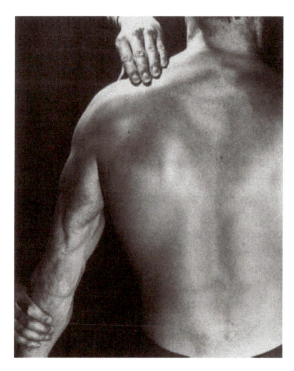

Fig. 4.9 Muscle: supraspinatus. Main segmental supply: C5. Peripheral nerve: suprascapula. Test: the patient tries to initiate abduction of the arm from the side against resistance. The first 30° of arm abduction.

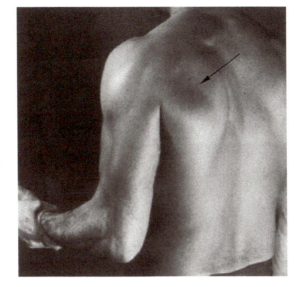

Fig. 4.10 Muscle: infraspinatus. Main segmental supply: C5. Peripheral nerve: suprascapular. Test: the patient flexes the elbow, holds the elbow to the side, and then attempts to externally rotate the forearm against resistance.

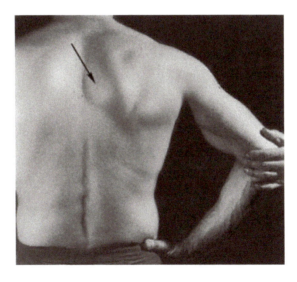

Fig. 4.11 Muscle: rhomboids. Main segmental supply: C5. Peripheral nerve: nerve to rhomboids. If the muscle is weak, the superior part of the scapular is abducted. Test: hand on hip, the patient tries to force the elbow backwards.

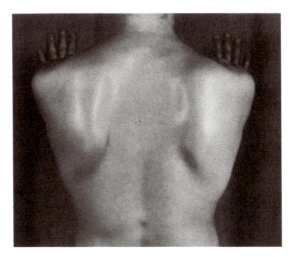

Fig. 4.12 Muscle: serratus anterior. Main segmental supply: C5–C7. Peripheral nerve: nerve to serratus anterior or the long thoracic nerve. If the muscle is weak, the tip of the scapula comes off the chest wall, the medial scapular border remains straight. Test: the patient pushes the arm forwards against firm obstruction.

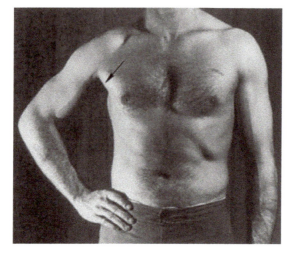

Fig. 4.13 Muscle: pectoralis major. Main segmental supply: C6–C8. Peripheral nerve: lateral and medial pectoral nerves. Test: placing the hand on the hip and pressing inwards, the sternocostal part of the muscle can be seen and felt to contract. Raising the arm forwards above 90° and attempting to adduct it against resistance brings the clavicular portion into action.

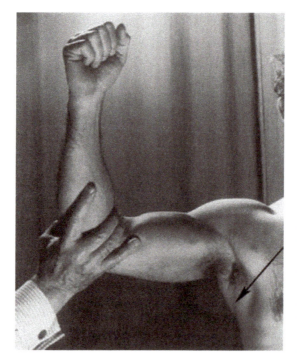
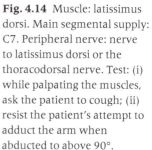

Fig. 4.14 Muscle: latissimus dorsi. Main segmental supply: C7. Peripheral nerve: nerve to latissimus dorsi or the thoracodorsal nerve. Test: (i) while palpating the muscles, ask the patient to cough; (ii) resist the patient's attempt to adduct the arm when abducted to above 90°.

Muscles of the elbow joint

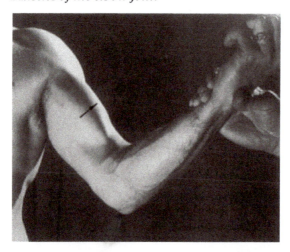

Fig. 4.15 Muscle: biceps. Main segmental supply: C5. Peripheral nerve: musculocutaneous. Test: the patient flexes the elbow against resistance, the forearm being supinated.

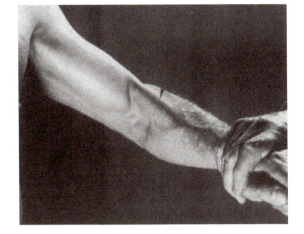

Fig. 4.16 Muscle: brachioradialis. Main segmental supply: C5, C6. Peripheral nerve: radial. Test: the patient pronates the forearm and draws the thumb towards the nose against resistance.

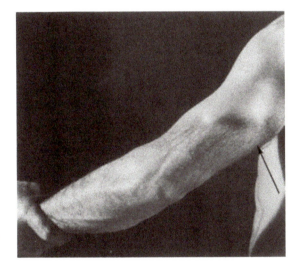

Fig. 4.17 Muscle: triceps. Main segmental supply: C7. Peripheral nerve: radial. Test: the patient attempts to extend the elbow against resistance.

Muscles of the forearm and wrist joint

Fig. 4.18 Muscle: extensor carpi radialis longus. Main segmental supply: C6, C7. Peripheral nerve: radial. Test: the patient holds the fingers partially extended and dorsiflexes the wrist towards the radial side against resistance.

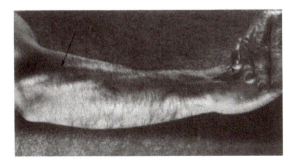

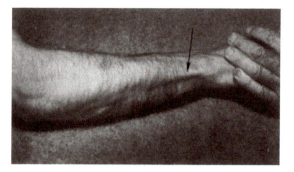

Fig. 4.19 Muscle: extensor carpis ulnaris. Main segmental supply: C7. Peripheral nerve: radial. Test: as Fig. 4.18, but dorsiflexion must be towards the ulnar side.

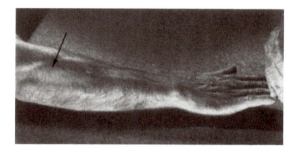

Fig. 4.20 Muscle: extensor digitorum. Main segmental supply: C7. Peripheral nerve: radial. Test: the examiner attempts to flex the patient's extended fingers at the metacarpophalangeal joints.

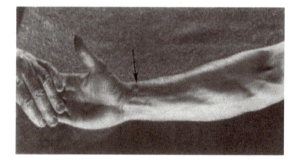

Fig. 4.21 Muscle: flexor carpi radialis. Main segmental supply: C6, C7. Peripheral nerve: median. Test: the examiner resists the patient's attempts to flex the wrist towards the radial side. Palmaris longus is also shown.

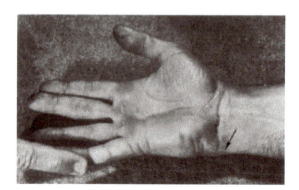

Fig. 4.22 Muscle: flexor carpi ulnaris. Main segmental supply: C8. Peripheral nerve: ulnar. Test: this muscle is best seen while testing the abductor digiti minimi, where it fixes its point of origin. Abduction of the thumb is the movement that brings the thumb to a right-angle with the palm. It is helpful if the patient's hand is held in the correct plane with the examiner's hand.

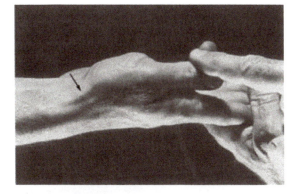

Fig. 4.23 Muscle: abductor pollicis longus. Main segmental supply: C8. Peripheral nerve: radial. Test: the patient attempts to maintain the thumb in abduction against the examiner's resistance.

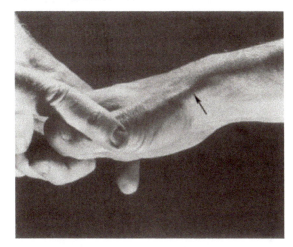

Fig. 4.24 Muscle: extensor pollicis brevis. Main segmental supply: C8. Peripheral nerve: radial. Test: the patient attempts to extend the thumb while the examiner attempts to flex it at the metacarpophalangeal joint.

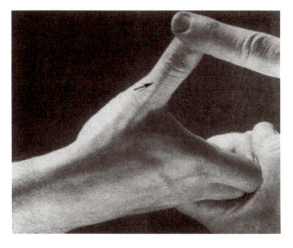

Fig. 4.25 Muscle: extensor pollicis longus. Main segmental supply: C8. Peripheral nerve: radial. Test: the patient attempts to extend the thumb while the examiner attempts to flex it at the interphalangeal joint.

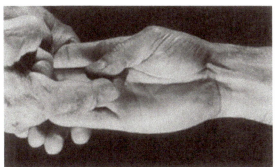

Fig. 4.26 Muscle: opponens pollicis. Main segmental supply: T1. Peripheral nerve: median. Test: the patient attempts to touch the little finger with the thumb. Preserved in ulnar nerve lesions when the rest of the hand appears very wasted.

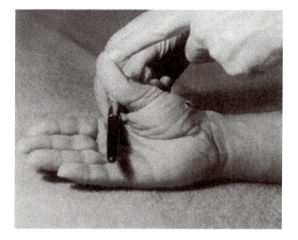

Fig. 4.27 Muscle: abductor pollicis brevis. Main segmental supply: T1. Peripheral nerve: median. Test: first place some object between the thumb and the base of the forefinger to prevent full adduction; then the patient attempts to raise the edge of the thumb vertically above the starting point, against resistance. This is an important muscle, being the first to show weakness in the common carpal tunnel syndrome.

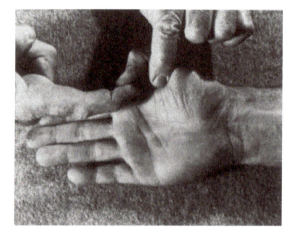

Fig. 4.28 Muscle: flexor pollicis longus. Main segmental supply: C8. Peripheral nerve: median. Test: the examiner attempts to extend the distal phalanx of the thumb against the patient's resistance. It is wise to hold the proximal phalanx.

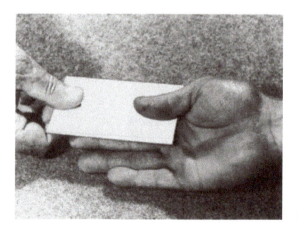

Fig. 4.29 Muscle: adductor pollicis. Main segmental supply: T1. Peripheral nerve: ulnar. Test: the patient attempts to hold a piece of paper between the thumb and the palmar aspect of the forefinger.

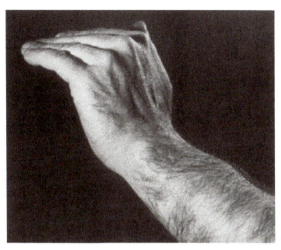

(a)

Fig. 4.30 Muscle: lumbricals and interossei. Main segmental supply: C8, T1. Peripheral nerve: median (lumbricals I and II); ulnar (interossei, lumbricals III and IV). Test: (a) the patient tries to flex the extended fingers at the metacarpophalangeal joints (lumbricals). (b) Next, the patient attempts to keep the fingers abducted against resistance (interossei).

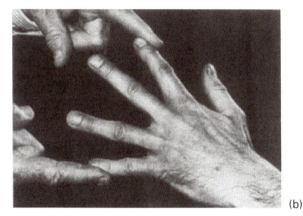

(b)

Fig. 4.31 Muscle: 1st dorsal interosseus and 1st palmar interosseus. Main segmental supply: T1. Peripheral nerve: ulnar. Test: place the hand flat on a table. The patient then tries to abduct (illustrated) and adduct the forefinger against resistance. This test can be applied to other fingers, but the muscles are not easily visible.

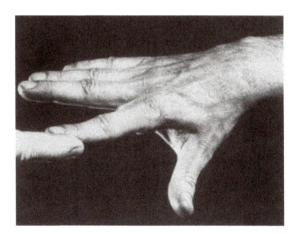

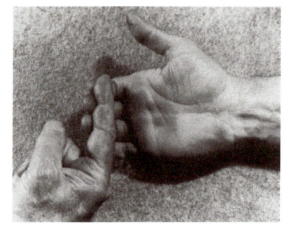

Fig. 4.32 Muscle: flexor digitorum sublimis. Main segmental supply: C8. Peripheral nerve: median. Test: the patient flexes the fingers at the proximal interphalangeal joint against resistance from the examiner's fingers placed on the middle phalanx.

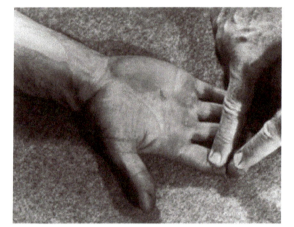

Fig. 4.33 Muscle: flexor digitorum profundus. Main segmental supply: C8. Peripheral nerve: median (I and II), ulnar (III and IV). Test: the patient flexes the terminal phalanx of the fingers against resistance, the middle phalanx being supported.

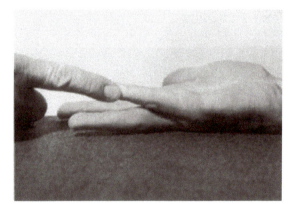

Fig. 4.34 Muscle: abductor digiti minimi. Main segmental supply: T1. Peripheral nerve: ulnar. Test: the back of the hand is placed on the table and the little finger abducted against resistance (see also Fig. 4.22). Often the only sign of an ulnar lesion.

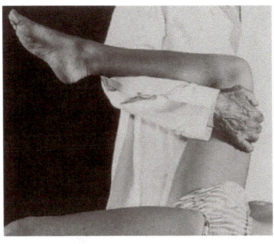

(a)

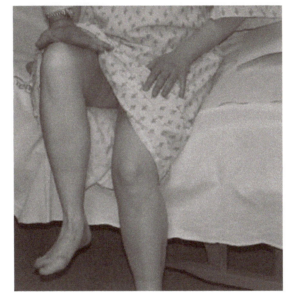

Fig. 4.35 (a) Muscle: ilipsoas. Main segmental supply L1–L3. Peripheral nerve: femoral. Test: the patient lies on the back and attempts to flex the thigh against resistance. Similarly, with the hip fully flexed, the patient resists attempts to extend it. (b) Iliopsoas testing. The patient resists the examiner's attempt to push the thigh to the bed.

(b)

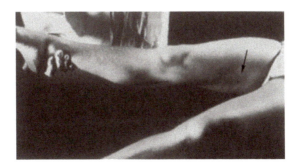

Fig. 4.36 Muscle: adductor femoris. Main segmental supply: L5, S1. Peripheral nerve: obdurator. Test: the patient attempts to adduct the leg against resistance.

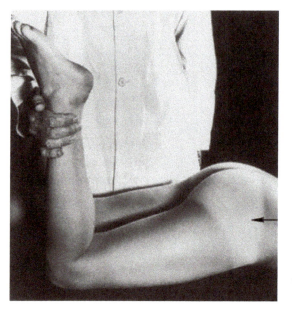

Fig. 4.37 Muscle: gluteus medius and minimus. Main segmental supply: L2, L3. Peripheral nerve: superior gluteal. Test: the patient, lying face down, flexes the knee and then forces the foot outwards against resistance. These muscles also abduct the extended leg.

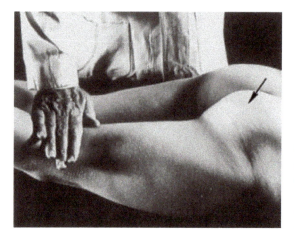

Fig. 4.38 Muscle: gluteus maximus. Main segmental supply: L5, S1. Peripheral nerve: inferior gluteal. Test: the patient, still lying on the stomach, should tighten the buttocks so that each can be palpated and compared; the patient must then try to raise the thigh against resistance. Important in caudal equina and conus medullaris lesions.

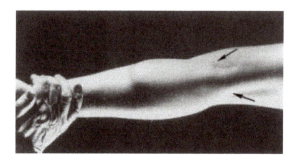

Fig. 4.39 Muscle: hamstrings (biceps, semitendinosus, semimembranosus). Main segmental supply: L4, L5, S1, S2. Peripheral nerve: sciatic. Test: the patient, lying on the stomach, attempts to flex the knee against resistance. The biceps is seen laterally, the semitendinosus medially.

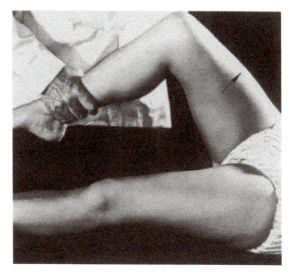

Fig. 4.40 Muscle: quadriceps femoris. Main segmental supply: L3, L4. Peripheral nerve: femoral. Test: the patient, lying on the back, attempts to extend the knee against resistance.

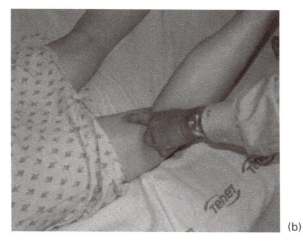

(a)

(b)

Fig. 4.41 (a) Muscle: semitendinosis. (b) Muscle: semimembranosus.

Muscles of the lower leg and ankle

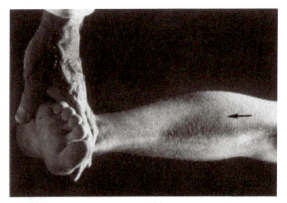

(a)

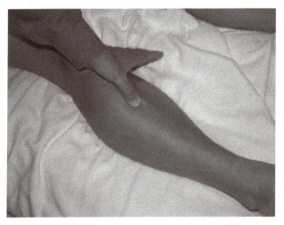

(b)

Fig. 4.42 The sciatic nerve divides into the medial and lateral popliteal nerves. The lateral popliteal further divides into anterior tibial and musculocutaneous branches. (a) Muscle: tibialis anticus. Main segmental supply: L4, L5. Peripheral nerve test: anterior tibial. Test: the patient dorsiflexes the foot against the resistance of the examiner's hand placed across the dorsum of the foot. (b) Test: the examiner compresses the muscle next to the tibial bone. Atrophy is easily appreciated.

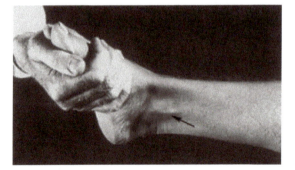

Fig. 4.43 Muscle: tibialis posticus. Main segmental supply: L4. Peripheral nerve: medial popliteal. Test: the patient plantar-flexes the foot slightly and then tries to invert it against resistance.

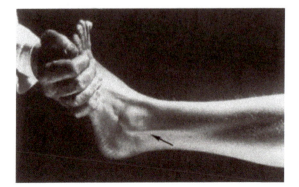

Fig. 4.44 Muscle: peronei. Main segmental supply: L5, S1. Peripheral nerve: musculocutaneous (principally). Test: the patient everts the foot against resistance. Isolated weakness may be the earliest sign of peroneal muscular atrophy.

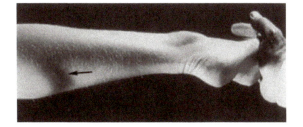

Fig. 4.45 Muscle: gastrocnemius. Main segmental supply: S1. Peripheral nerve: medial popliteal. Test: the patient plantar-flexes against resistance.

Muscles of the foot and great toe

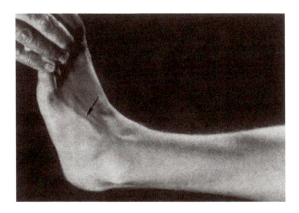

Fig. 4.46 Muscle: extensor digitorum longus. Main segmental supply: L5. Peripheral nerve: anterior tibial. Test: the patient dorsiflexes the toes against resistance.

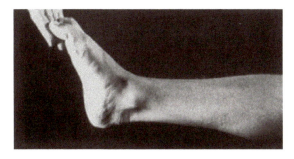

Fig. 4.47 Muscle: flexor digitorum longus. Main segmental supply: S1, S2. Peripheral nerve: medial popliteal. Test: the patient flexes the terminal phalanges against resistance.

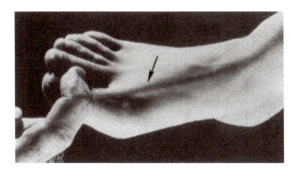

Fig. 4.48 Muscle: extensor hallucis. Main segmental supply: L5, S1. Peripheral nerve: anterior tibial. Test: the patient attempts to dorsiflex the great toe against resistance.

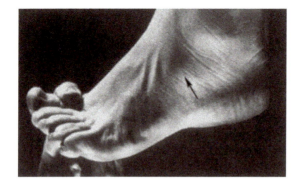

Fig. 4.49 Muscle: extensor digitorum brevis. Main segmental supply: S1. Peripheral nerve: anterior tibial. Test: the patient dorsiflexes the great toe against resistance. The triangular muscle is an example of an S1 innervated muscle. If atrophied, the examiner has a direct objective view of the root.

(a)

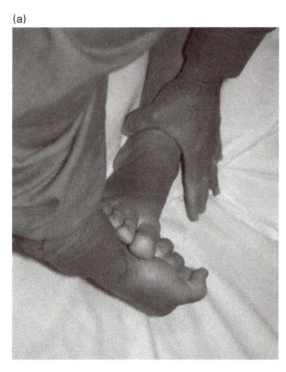

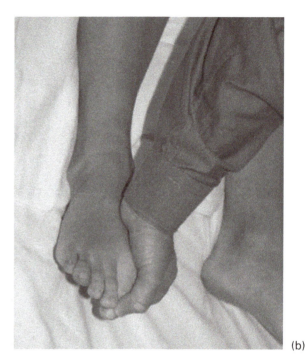

(b)

(c)

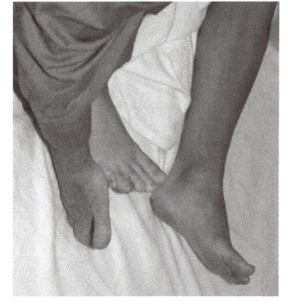

Fig. 4.50 (a) The patient's foot is placed in abduction against the examiner's hand. The patient is then asked to adduct the foot against resistance. The L4 root and the posterior tibial nerve are tested. (b) extensor hallices longus (EHL) – leveraged. The patient attempts to extend the great toe after it has been placed in flexion. An extremely sensitive evaluation of the L5 root. The examiner concomitantly carefully re-evaluates for atrophy along the tibia. (c) The examiner places the foot in adduction and then asks the patient to bring it to the midline. This is extremely sensitive for evaluating the S1 root. If a patient can abduct the little toe on one side but cannot on the other, this is further confirmation of S1 root weakness.

Types of muscle weakness

Weakness resulting from corticospinal tract lesions

Lesions of the corticospinal pathways from the motor cortex to the anterior horn cell are most often incomplete and affect particular groups of muscles and movements rather than individual muscles. Weakness is noted in the abductors and extensors of the upper extremity and the extensor of the thumb is particularly important to evaluate if the lesion is suspected to be at a cortical level. The exact location of the innervation of the hand has been identified and is noted as the "motor knuckle" (area 4). This area of the cortex is frequently affected by an embolus to the centrosulcal branch of the superior division of the middle cerebral artery. Patients present with a dropped wrist that appears to be a radial palsy (a pseudoradial palsy). Finger flexors are involved, which distinguishes it from a true radial palsy in which they are not.

The ability to perform individual fractionated movements of the fingers and toes is characteristic of an intact pyramidal system. If it is lesioned, all fingers move together. An exception is a lesion in the ventral pons in which proximal muscles are affected and distal muscles of the upper extremity are spared. Corticospinal lesions show distal greater than proximal weakness and are associated with spasticity, a hemiplegic gait and Babinski's sign. They demonstrate a fix on arm roll, drift of both arm and leg and the shortening response (Fig. 4.51–4.54).

Weakness resulting from extrapyramidal lesions

There is no actual loss of strength with extrapyramidal lesions, but there is an abnormality of tone and the ability to sustain an initiated movement. There is dysregulation of tone so that the agonist muscle has to move the joints of the limb against the resistance of an antagonist muscle. If the patient is asked to sustain finger movement, it is noted that each preprogrammed movement gets smaller and smaller. A patient with Parkinson's disease will frequently complain that he or she cannot sign a full signature. Each letter becomes smaller and smaller and the end of the last name is almost a straight line. Initiation of movement is slow. The increased tone affects the whole limb and is associated with rigidity and generally decreased reflexes. There are fewer spontaneous and associated movements.

Weakness resulting from lower motor neuron disease

This form of weakness is marked and if from pure anterior horn cell disease is often associated with atrophy and fasciculations. Viral illness such as polio or other neurotrophic viruses may affect individual anterior horn cells, so that weakness is asymmetrical and may involve individual small

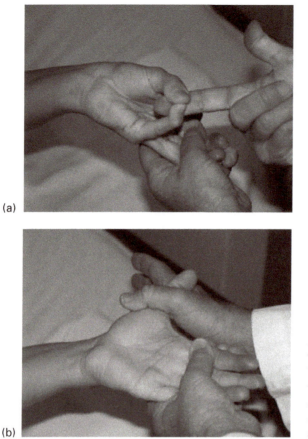

(a)

(b)

Fig. 4.51 The patient is opposing the oppens pollicis and the oppens digiti quinti. The examiner is attempting to break the locked ring. Subtle weakness can be better appreciated by placing the oppen pollicis in maximal abduction.

muscle groups such as the intrinsic hand muscles. One or two lumbricales or one extensor muscle would be involved in this instance. If the process affects only the anterior horn cells such as occurs with hereditary motor neuron disease (progressive spinal muscle atrophy), wasting is prominent in the end and tends to be symmetrical while reflexes are lost. ALS in general is asymmetrical. There is wasting of muscle in the presence of hyperactive reflexes. A lesion of the ventral root affects those muscles whose sole or major supply is from that segment. A common example of this process is seen with the prominent deltoid wasting of severe cervical spondylosis often with induced or spontaneous fasciculations ("spondylitic ALS"). If the peripheral nerve is lesioned (e.g., sciatic), all muscles supplied by that nerve are affected. Motor neuropathies that are dying back (metabolic, toxic and occasionally genetic) show maximal weakness peripherally and symmetrically in the arm and legs. Autoimmune peripheral neuropathies may be asymmetrical and affect the upper extremities prior to the lower (GM1 neuropathy or multifocal neuropathy with conduction block).

Weakness resulting from muscular lesions

In most acquired inflammatory myopathies the weakness is proximal.

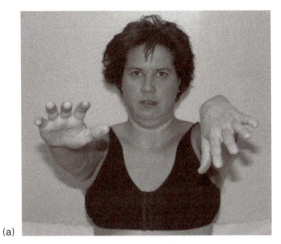

(a)

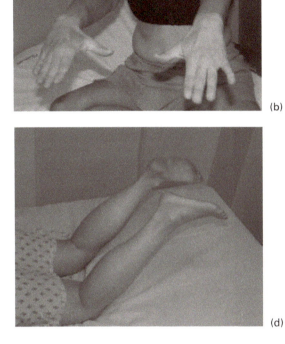

(b)

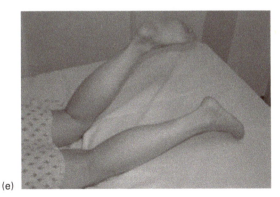

(c)

(d)

(e)

Fig. 4.52 (a) Extensor drift. Note that the left thumb is adducted and the wrist drops. Could also be a pseudoradial palsy from a motor knuckle lesion. (b) The fifth finger cannot remain adducted and drifts outward (Alter's sign). (c) Lengthening test. The patient is asked to fully extend and flex the arm. The side opposite the corticospinal tract lesion does not fully extend. (d) Leg drift. Normal leg position. (e) Leg drift. Weakness and downward drift of the left leg from a right corticospinal lesion.

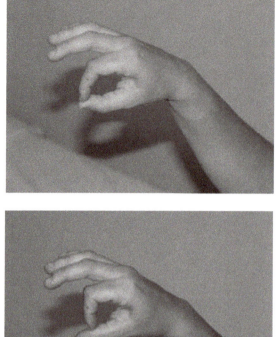

(a)

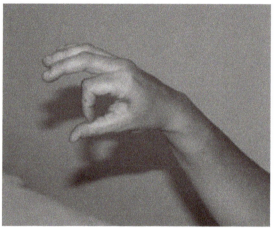

(b)

Fig. 4.53 (a) Pyramidal movement. The corticospinal track most often functions at the tips of the finger. Facility, rhythm and maintenance of movement are noted. (b) Fine movement performed at the distal interphalangeal crease. This is an unusual position and movement is not performed as well. Observe the speed and facility of the movement. A more sensitive way to evaluate pyramidal movement.

The exception is inclusion body myositis (IBM) which affects forearm flexors with associated contracture of finger flexors. Hereditary IBM may specifically target the distal quadriceps. The distal genetic myopathies affect the anterior or posterior compartments of the lower legs (Welander's, Miyoshi's, Markesberry/Griggs/Udd) or the sternocleidomastoids, masseter and distal extremity (myotonic dystrophy type I).

Local injury or compartment syndromes may affect the specific muscles of that compartment. In nerve or root lesions, the muscles that are affected are those of a specific nerve or spinal segment. There may be wasting, pseudohypertrophy or tenderness. The related reflexes are depressed or lost.

Myasthenia gravis

Specific muscle groups may be affected. There is an ocular form alone and a primary bulbar form. Characteristically, in generalized myasthenia, the degree of weakness varies with time, increases with use, but recovers with rest often after a short period of time. Myasthenic weakness is most frequently seen in the eyelids, the external ocular muscles, the tongue (triple furrowed tongue), the throat and larynx, the muscles of the back, shoulder and hand. Cogan's twitch sign demonstrates subtle weakness of the

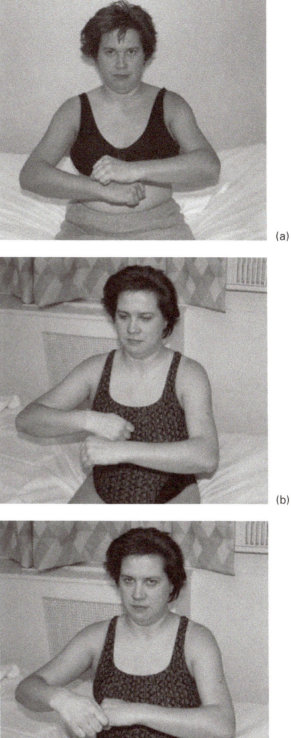

(a)

(b)

Fig. 4.54 (a) Arm roll. The patient rotates one arm over the other. The arm that does not roll as well is opposite the side of a corticospinal lesion. (b) Note the right arm rotating around the fixed left arm. (c) The arm roll is also excellent to discern the affected side in Parkinson's disease or other akinetic-rigid syndromes.

(c)

superior rectus and inferior oblique muscles. The patient is asked to maintain up gaze for 20–30 seconds which fatigues the superior rectus and inferior oblique muscles. The patient is asked to follow the examiner's finger below the horizontal and back to the horizontal. The lids will be seen to rise above the iris and then settle to their normal position. The law of equal innervation for yoked muscles (Hitzig's law) states that muscles that work in tandem receive equal innervation. If the superior rectus and inferior oblique are fatigued in up gaze, they receive maximal innervation. This increases the innervation to the levator palebral muscle (yoked muscle) which causes the upper lid to retract away (increased lid retraction) from the iris on up gaze (more than is necessary) and then settle to normal position (a Cogan's twitch).

If a patient with possible myasthenic weakness gets stronger with exercise, one should suspect Lambert–Eaton myasthenic syndrome from small cell cancer of the lung. In general, with Lambert–Eaton syndrome ptosis is more common than extraocular muscle weakness, the legs are weaker than the arms and there is a "load in the pants" gait. The autonomic nervous system is affected from the autoimmune attack and patients complain of a dry mouth and inability to swallow.

Cholinergic crisis

The treatment of myasthenia gravis has dramatically improved with the use of immunosuppression, intravenous immunoglobulin (IVIG) and plasmapheresis. It is rare to see patients on very large doses of anticholinesterase agents. A cholinergic crisis is suspected in a myasthenic patient with increasing weakness, hyperhidrosis, constricted pupils, hyperactive bowel sounds and bradycardia.

Hysterical weakness

The overwhelming majority of patients that are seen in clinic have real disease. The bias of the examiner should always be that the patient has organic disease. Some patients feel the need to "catastrophize" and exaggerate their problem in the face of organic disease. Their weakness often varies in degree and distribution, has a "give way" quality to it, and does not correspond to a root, nerve or pyramidal distribution.

Posture, stance, spinal movement and gait (Fig. 4.55)

The most informative time to observe the patient's gait and station is when he or she does not realize they are being watched. This occurs at the end of the examination when leaving the office. It is often instructive to watch the patient go through a door (difficult for a Parkinson's disease or basal ganglia patient) because of the need to change motor programs.

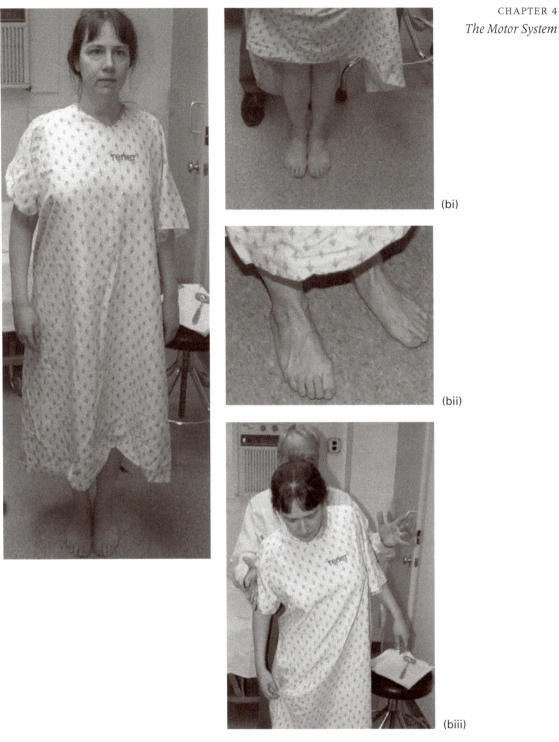

(bi)

(bii)

(a)

(biii)

Fig. 4.55 (a) Romberg test. Patient stands with feet together and eyes open and maintains the stance without sway. (b) As soon as the patient closes her eyes, she sways more than normally and then breaks stance. A positive test. (*Cont'd on page 122*).

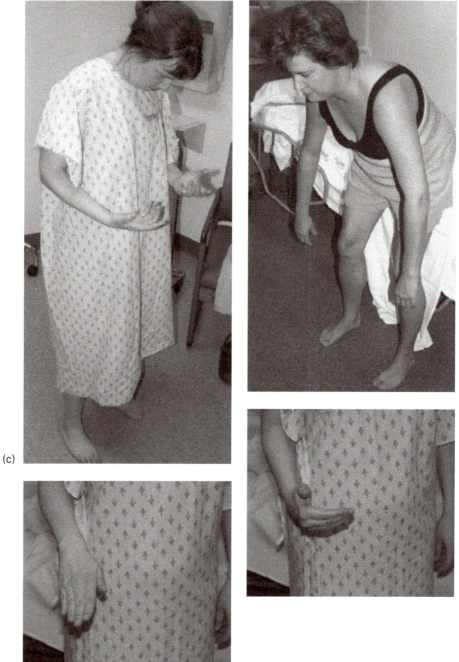

Fig. 4.55 (*cont'd*) (c) Basal ganglia posture. Head and body flexion; increased carrying angles of the arms; metacarpophalangeal flexion of the hands; broad base. (d) Simian posture of spinal stenosis. Note the straight lower back and hanging arms. (e) Cortical adducted thumb; corticospinal disease. (f) Metacarpophalangeal flexion of basal ganglia disease.

Posture and stance

The patient is evaluated standing with the great toe and heels touching. The patient is observed to detect unnatural sway or if he or she breaks stance and has to step off to maintain balance. The maneuver is evaluated with the eyes opened and closed. The patient is asked to turn and equilibrium during the maneuver is evaluated. Inability to stand with the feet together suggests cerebellar, dorsal column or vestibular disease. Breaking stance with eyes closed suggests dorsal column disease. Vestibular patients immediately broaden their base with eye closure.

The Back (Fig. 4.56)

This is often the most important part of the examination both for back

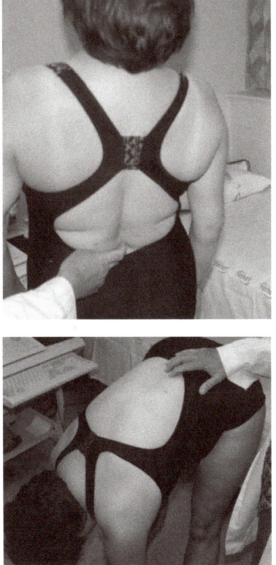

(a)

(b)

Fig. 4.56 (a) Evaluation for scoliosis and increased lordosis at L4–L5. Each interspace is palpated as the affected one is often painful. (b) Flexion and extension cause pain at the involved segment. Note the conversion of lordosis to a smooth curve. (*Cont'd on* *page 124*).

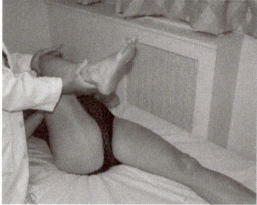

(c)

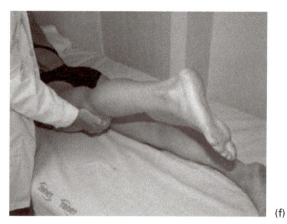

(f)

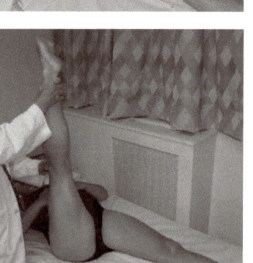

(d)

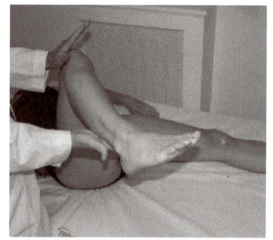

(gi)

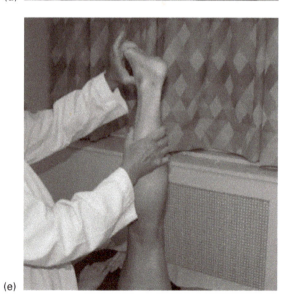

(e)

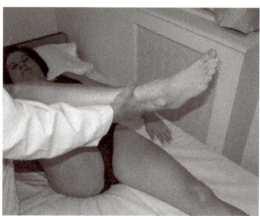

(gii)

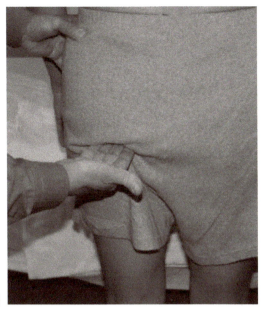

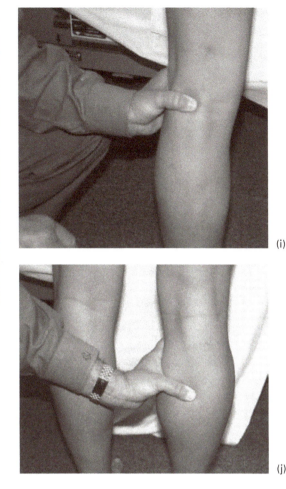

(h)

(i)

(j)

Fig. 4.56 (c) Straight leg raising (SLR). The thigh is brought to the abdomen, which is rarely painful. (d) The leg is extended on the abdomen. The hamstrings will go into spasm and the patient will complain of pain if the sciatic nerve is compressed by pathology or is sensitized. (e) Lasègue's maneuver. The foot is flexed downward with the leg extended. This produces pain in the sciatic nerve if it is sensitized. (f) Reverse SLR test. The patient lies flat on the abdomen and the leg is extended. There will be pain at L4–L5 with spinal stresses and the groin will be sore under the inguinal ligament if the femoral nerve is sensitized. (gi) The leg is externally and internally rotated. If there is hip pathology, there will be pain in the hip joint itself. (gii) External rotation of the leg. If internal and external rotation do not cause pain and the hip hurts, it is probably referred pain from the L5 root. (h) Compression of the sciatic notch which depolarizes the sciatic nerve itself or its sensitized nervi-nervorum from a higher lesion. (i) Compression of the common peroneal and anterior tibial nerve in the posterior popliteal fossa which if sensitized is painful. (j) Compression of the gastrocnemius muscle is painful because of sensitization of deep muscle afferents from a higher level lesion (disk at L5–S1).

pathology as well as leg pain. The patient is examined for lordosis, kyphosis and scoliosis. Patients with an abnormally deep lordotic curve at L4–L5 frequently have abnormal stretch of nerve roots at that level. A pelvic tilt is often seen with spondylolisthesis. The roots contralateral to the convexity of a scoliosis have to travel a greater distance to their exit foramina and may be under tension. The patient is asked to touch the toes. Mechanical back disease of almost any sort limits flexion and extension. The alignment of the spinous processes, the conversion of lordosis to a smooth curve is noted. Patients with mechanical back disease from L4–S1 have particular difficulty with extension. Lateral movement and flexion is observed. Paraspinal muscle spasm is caused by abnormal afferent pain barrages at the appropriate level that trigger muscle contraction from pain barrages exciting anterior horn cells and not from damage to the muscle or ligament. The thumb is used to elicit tenderness between the spinous process which is an excellent objective sign of segmental back disease. If weakness of back muscles is suspected, the patient is asked to squat and then stand. In normal patients, the back is straight. Percussion of the spinous processes often elicits pain if there is deep bone pathology (particularly cancer and infection).

5: Posture, Stance and Spinal Movement

Abnormalities of posture, stance and spinal movement

Bradykinesia

This physical sign is characteristic of Parkinson's disease and all akinetic rigid syndromes. The movement is slow, its initiation is delayed, and there are no or minimal spontaneous movements. Normal eye blinks are 14 per minute. A bradykinetic patient may blink less than seven times a minute, which frequently simulates a serpentine stare. There is difficulty and decreased turning in bed. Spouses complain that the patient is in the same position in bed in which they went to sleep. Patients have difficulty in changing motor programs. This is often noted when passing through a doorway. The patient freezes and then utilizes small cautious steps to change direction.

A stooped position (Fig. 5.1)

In diseases of the basal ganglia, the patient has flexed truncal posture, increased flexion of the arms and a forward flexed head. If the head is extended and the nasolabial folds are deep with flexed arms, the patient has progressive supranuclear palsy. The hands are flexed at the metacarpophalangeal joint in all basal ganglia disease. As Professor Spillane notes*, "Patients that are tall, old, have poor muscular development and overbearing relatives may have stooped posture." The head may fall forward on the chest in severe motor neuron disease, myasthenia gravis and polymyositis. All elderly patients have a forward flexed neck resulting from cervical spondylosis ("spondylitic neck posture") caused by arthritic degeneration of the uncovertebral joints and desiccation of the cervical disks. If this process is severe, the examiner must be aware that it will be associated with:
1 inability to tandem walk (compression of the laterally placed dorsal and ventral spinocerebellar tracts);
2 an inverted radial or supinator reflex at C5–C6;
3 hyperactive knee jerks.
Compression of the cervical spine from spondylosis or stenosis dramatically affects other parts of the neurologic examination, particularly the reflexes.

* Bickerstaff's Neurological Examination in Clinical Practice, 6th Edition, John Spillane, Blackwell Publishing, Oxford, 1996.

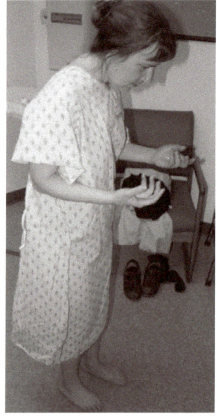

(a)

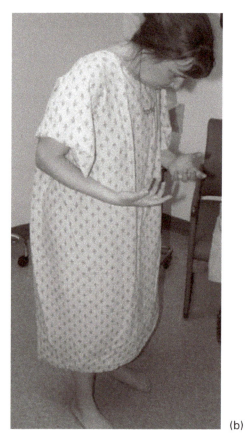

(b)

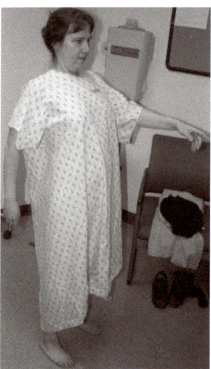

(c)

Fig. 5.1 (a) Normal pressure
hydrocephalus (NPH) with forward flexed
posture, increased carrying angle of the
arms with a normal base. (b) Parkinsonian
shuffling, broad-based gait; stance is
increased. (c) Martinette gait of alcoholic
patient with anterior vermis degeneration.
Patients have an extended spine.

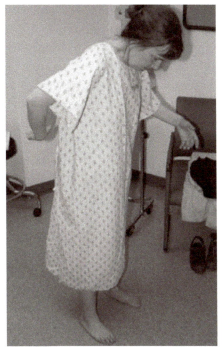

(e)

(d)

Fig. 5.1 (*cont'd*) (d) Parietal gait. The patient cautiously advances the foot on the side without neglect. (e) Thalamic gait. The patient is unaware of the wandering of the right arm from lack of position sense.

Kyphoscoliosis

A kyphotic spine is common with aging and severe emphysema. It may be so extreme in ankylosing spondylitis that the patient may not be able to lift the head above the horizontal. It also is associated with the human leukocyte antigen (HLA) antigen B27 and a brittle cervical spine.

Scoliosis may be divided into C and S forms. The former is noted with acquired disease such as a syrinx tumor or hemangioma. These processes cause denervation of the paraspinal muscles on one side. This may be seen in children with a long-standing spinal cord astrocytoma. Astrocytomas may also occur in the walls of a syrinx. The S form has a compensatory cervical curve and is often hereditary. Scoliosis is a common marker of hereditary cerebellar ataxia (Friedreich's) and neuropathy. It is invariant in late-stage muscle disease particularly Duchenne's and Becker's muscular dystrophy as well as von Recklinghausen's disease (type I chromosome 17).

Severe kyphoscoliosis may cause spinal cord compression and paraplegia. The latter may occur during surgical procedures to correct the scoliosis.

129

This complication is now avoided by evoked potential monitoring while the patient is under anesthesia.

Lumbar disk disease irritates the ipsilateral ventral roots with chronic muscle contraction and produces scoliosis to the side of the lesion. It is maximal at the affected level and increases with flexion. Congenital hemivertebrar causes extreme scoliosis on forward flexion. Usually, 12° of scoliosis is cause for concern.

Disk disease in conjunction with scoliosis is often symptomatic and complicates normal alignment because the root opposite the convexity is under tension. Hemivertebrae or maldeveloped vertebrae may be associated with disk disease and other congenital abnormalities at the level of the scoliosis.

Excessive lordosis

This is characteristic in some ethnic groups and is often asymptomatic. It is common in many congenital myopathies and is particularly prominent in Duchenne's and Becker's muscular dystrophy. It is occasionally seen in severe myasthenia gravis and congenital hip disease.

A rigid spine

This is common in specific muscle diseases:
1 type II fiber type disproportion;
2 Emery–Dreifuss muscular dystrophy;
3 a few patients with fascioscapular humeral (FSH) muscular dystrophy;
4 myofibrillar myopathy;
5 limb girdle muscular dystrophy (LGMD 2).
In ankylosing spondylitis, the entire spine moves en bloc and flexion only occurs at the hip joints. The lumbar spine may remain straight on flexion from paravertebral spasm from any cause.

A tender spine

Local bony tumors including osteoid osteomas, articular bone cysts and hemangiomas cause local tenderness on percussion. Incredible pain is caused by diskitis. Just touching a patient's bed causes extreme pain and should suggest this diagnosis in a patient who has recently had a spinal operation or who is an intravenous drug abuser. Epidural pus and blood cause tenderness and spasm over many segments. Epidural catheters for bupivacaine anesthesia and patients who are being anticoagulated are at risk for these complications.

Abnormalities of equilibrium

Inability to remain upright occurs with large lesions of the cerebellar vermis and the fourth ventricle. This postural instability is out of proportion to limb ataxia or any ataxia with the patient recumbent. Falling backwards is characteristic of all basal ganglia disease, normal pressure hydrocephalus, progressive supranuclear palsy and acquired hepatolenticular degeneration.

Vestibular diseases cause the patient to feel as if they are pushed to one side (lateral pulsion). This can occur with both pure lesions of the labyrinth or from destruction of the vestibular pathways in the brainstem. If a patient feels he or she is being pushed or falls forward this is characteristic of otolith antigravity utriculus and sacculus disease. Patients with hemispheric cerebellar disease fall to the side of the lesion.

Basilar invagination occurs when the odontoid process rises above Chamberlain's line. This is a line drawn from the back of the hard palate to the inner table of the occipital bone. If the odontoid is 2–3 mm above this line it compresses the brainstem particularly when the head is extended. In Arnold–Chiari malformation the cerebellar tonsils descend and compress the dorsal part of the brainstem. Any increase of intraspinal pressure from coughing, sneezing or even extending the head can further compress the medullary pyramids and the patient loses all tone in the legs and collapses.

Positive Romberg test (see Fig. 4.55)

The test depends on the integrity of proprioception from the joints of the legs. The patient stands with the feet (great toe and heels opposed). This is accomplished with minimal sway, but the patient does not break stance. If the eyes are closed and there is significant proprioceptive deficit, the patient breaks stance to broaden the base. A positive Romberg occurs with high cervical cord compression from stenosis or cervical spondylosis, tabes dorsalis, B_{12} deficiency, HIV (cervical myelopathy) and, rarely, Sjögren's syndrome. It occurs with autoimmune lesions of the dorsal root ganglia.

Squatting and standing up

Weakness of the proximal leg and paraspinal muscles makes it impossible to get out of a squat position. Patients employ Gower's maneuver (climbing up the legs) to push themselves up by placing their hands at higher levels on the legs. This is most clearly seen in the muscular dystrophies, but occurs in proximal lower extremity weakness from polymyositis, peripheral neuropathy or myasthenia gravis.

Gait (see Fig. 5.1)

Almost all central and peripheral nervous system diseases have a characteristic gait. An excellent way to evaluate all aspects of gait is to follow the patient into the examination room after the history taking. Patients are unaware that they are being formally examined and are at their most natural. An astute examiner should be close to the diagnosis by evaluating gait properly. Of course, the astute history taker already has the diagnosis and is performing the examination to prove it. The stamping gait of the patient with tabes dorsalis is no longer heard (although it may make a comeback in conjunction with HIV), but certainly the slapping gait of peroneal palsy and that of peripheral neuropathy will be with us.

The examiner notes gait ignition, the carrying angle and movement of the arms, the stride length and the smoothness of movement, the distance the legs are apart, the ability to maintain a straight line and to turn without stepping off. The examiner should be able to determine which component of the central or peripheral nervous system is affected.

Abnormalities of gait

Dragging the feet

This is usually a result of hemiplegia of any cause. The patient cannot lift the leg high enough to clear the floor because of weakness of the iliopsoas and the anterior tibialis muscles. The abductors of the hip are substituted to tilt the pelvis of the affected side upwards. This is called a circumducting gait. The arm is flexed across the body and if the process is severe the patient will abduct and circumduct it as well. In repose the foot will be inverted and dropped.

If the patient has bilateral upper motor lesions (usually brainstem strokes or head injury), both feet do not clear the floor and drag, the legs are stiff and the steps are small, the patient leans forward. If the process is congenital or acquired in early childhood (placental stroke or *in utero* brain injury), there is adduction, hypertonicity and spasm. This leads to a scissor component of the gait which causes the legs to cross. This may also be accompanied by calf muscle contracture with consequent toe walking.

High-stepping gait

The foot is raised high above the ground because of weakness of the anterior tibialis and foot extensors. The toe hits the ground first. The patient flexes the hip and knee to raise the foot. He or she is not ataxic. If unilateral, it is caused by peroneal nerve palsy or an L4–L5 lesion that paralyzes the anterior tibialis muscle. It is most common bilaterally from hereditary sensory motor neuropathies (pes cavus, loss of all muscles below the knee, distal one-third of the quadriceps atrophy), cauda equina lesions, distal myopathies with anterior compartment atrophy (Welander, Laing, Markesberry/Udd/Griggs variants), scapuloperoneal syndromes, and most commonly in severe autoimmune neuropathies (Guillain–Barré syndrome (GBS)). A painless foot drop may also herald amyotrophic lateral sclerosis (ALS).

If position sense is severely affected from destruction of the large proprioceptive neurons of the dorsal root ganglia (autoimmune disorders,

Richter's variant of GBS, paraneoplastic antibody attack, Sjögren's syndrome, sarcoid) or cisplatinum, the patient is unaware of the position of the feet. The foot and leg may flail side to side, the base is wide, the heel strikes the ground first and there is often a similar picture occurring in the upper extremities. The patient may not be able to walk in the dark as visual compensation is lost (sensory ataxia).

A shuffling gait (see Fig. 5.1)

This is the gait of a severe parkinsonian patient, but occurs in any basal ganglia disease. There is frequently gait ignition failure. The patient has a hard time taking the first step. The patient is forward flexed; the carrying angles of the arm are increased in flexion. The patient shuffles the feet and slides them along the ground in a flat-footed manner. Bradykinesia and rigidity are evident with concomitant flexion of the hips and knees. As the patient moves, the steps become more rapid (festination) as if the patient is trying to maneuver the body over the center of gravity. Lack of associated arm movement is evident and often asymmetrical. The patient has difficulty stopping and maintaining position if gently pushed forward (propulsion). He or she is unable to easily pass through a doorway and stops with a series of small steps (inability to change motor programs). This problem may sometimes be avoided by visual fixation on an object or crack in the floor beyond the doorway.

A small-stepped shuffling gait is seen in normal pressure hydrocephalus (NPH). The patient may have gait ignition failure (foot grasp of the floor) or raise and lower the feet in the same place ("egg walking"), this is apraxia of gait. The patient frequently falls backwards. In multi-infarct states (status lacunaire), usually from small vessel disease, the patient has a shuffling small-stepped gait that is irregular and hesitant ("marche a petite pas").

An ataxic gait

A lateral cerebellar hemisphere lesion causes the patient to be unsteady and fall to the ipsilateral side. The base is wide, the leg moves irregularly when flexed and extended and the patient sways and rocks to that side. If there is bilateral hemispheric cerebellar disease, the patient has a broad base, rocks and sways from side to side. The back is straight if the vermis is uninvolved.

Ataxia of the trunk is caused by midline vermian lesions. The patient when sitting has lost extensor tone of the paraspinal muscles and titubates (sways). If the arms are outstretched, the drift is upwards. The patient is completely unstable when standing, reels in all directions including backwards and needs support to walk. Vermian lesions are caused by cerebellar hemorrhage, tumors, demyelinating disease and compression from tonsillar descent into the foramen magnum.

An anterior cerebellar gait occurs from lesions of the anterior vermis (the lingula, culmen and centralis) is most often seen in severe alcoholism.

The patient has a stiff-legged extensor posture and tends to lean backwards ("martinette gait") (see Fig. 5.1).

Severely affected multiple sclerosis patients demonstrate truncal and vermian ataxia with vertical oscillation of the head and spasticity. Many heredofamilial spastic-ataxic syndromes are similar, but lack the head oscillations and characteristic eye findings that are seen in multiple sclerosis.

A waddling gait

This is seen in muscle disease or any illness that weakens the iliopsoas muscles. The patient utilizes the gluteus medius and minimus muscles to lift and rotate the pelvis to compensate for inability to flex the iliopsoas muscle. The patient may also utilize upper trunk muscles in this compensation. The congenital myopathies and muscular dystrophies demonstrate this gait. The gait is also seen with congenital dislocation of the hip.

Hysterical gait

These were described extensively in soldiers from the trenches of World War I. They were designated astasia-abasia. Hysterical gaits are bizarre, do not conform to any known pattern of weakness or pathology, differ from examination to examination, do not cause injury and may disappear when the patient thinks he or she is not observed. The bias of the examiner should be that there is an underlying problem. The patient is exaggerating disability to gain the attention of the examiner.

The gait in chorea

Huntington's chorea is characterized by a lurching gait that is wide based, reeling from heel to heel with variable steps and associated with vigorous grimace and movements of the hands and wrist. Choreatic eye movements are prominent. In Sydenham's and other choreas, arms, neck and face movements are prominent with walking, but the gait itself is minimally involved. The dyskinesias induced by dopaminergic drugs commonly affect the shoulder, face and extremities more than the gait. There is no lurching quality. In central dystonias the patient may walk on the everted foot, although normal foot posture can be accomplished in recumbency. In peripheral dystonia from chronic regional pain syndrome, the patient walks on the sole. In repose the foot is dropped and inverted.

Minor abnormalities

Elderly patients may have severe cervical spondylosis with consequent loss of proprioception from the legs. As we age we lose dopaminergic cells in a linear manner from the pars compacta of the substantia nigra. We all start a parkinsonian posture with a forward flexed neck and upper body. Our steps will become slightly shorter. If we continue from minimal cognitive impairment (word-finding difficulties and slight slowness of processing) to frank organic brain syndrome, our gait will be cautious and slightly broad based (a Wells' dementia gait). Normal aging brings with it loss of vibration and proprioceptive disability in the lower extremities which adds to unsteadiness and falls.

Minor abnormalities of gait are easily demonstrated by asking the patient to walk heel to toe both forwards and backwards. Patients with cerebellar lesions fall to the side of the lesion. Generalized proprioceptive deficits cause the patient to fall to either side. If a patient is asked to circle a chair in alternate directions, a right cerebellar hemispheric lesion causes the patient to bump into the chair on the right; on circling the chair to the left the patient will deviate away from it. A patient with a cerebellar lesion cannot stand unaided or hop on one foot. A normal person can hop up and down at least three times without difficulty. The heel does not touch the floor unless there is weakness.

6: Involuntary Movements

In evaluating the patient with involuntary movements, the examiner must discern the following:

1 What part(s) of the body are affected?
2 Is it constant or intermittent?
3 Is it present at rest, intention or both?
4 Does voluntary movement increase or suppress it?
5 Is it altered by any position of the limbs or trunk?
6 Is it affected by the environment, temperature or the patient's emotional state?
7 Is it suppressed or exaggerated by visual input?
8 Occurrence during sleep?
9 Is the patient conscious of it and, if so, can they suppress it?

A great deal of the examination occurs while the history is taken. The examiner should note the position of the patient in the chair. Patients with cerebellar disease, particularly the vermis, utilize the back of the chair for support. Basal ganglia disease patients are rigid and forward flexed. The choreoathetotic movements of Huntington's disease and peak dose dyskinesias of dopaminergic therapy in Parkinson's disease are evident. A side-to-side head tremor suggests essential tremor, an up and down oscillation of the head, a third ventricular tumor in a child or basal ganglia disease in an adult. A dropped and plantar flexed foot, suggests the dystonia of chronic regional pain syndrome (CRPS) or a primary dystonia. Tremor at rest indicates Parkinson's disease. Generalized rigidity, stiff person's syndrome, an akinetic rigid syndrome (multiple system atrophy (MSA), corticobasal ganglionic degeneration, frontal temporal degeneration (FTD)-chromosome 17 parkinsonism), tics and vocalizations, with abnormal movements suggest Tourette's disease, and startle myoclonus (myriachit, the "jumping Frenchmen" of Quebec). There is a genetic deficit of glycine, an inhibitory spinal cord neurotransmitter.

There is no other aspect of neurology that requires as good a clinical examination as that for involuntary movement. The good examiner trumps all imaging devices in most instances within 2–3 seconds. There is no magnetic resonance imaging (MRI) abnormality in most patients with Parkinson's disease.

The patient is then observed as he or she walks to the examining room. The specific gait abnormality is noted. Motor overflow of the arms and fingers are observed as is the position of the arm during associated movement. The patient is asked to hold the arms in front and specific drifts and hand postures are noted. The patient is then asked to hold the hands above the head with the palms forward (in dystonias and choreoathetotic states the hands, arms and shoulders will rotate). The patient is asked to perform the finger to nose test and hold the arms steadily flexed in front (the former cerebellar function and the latter demonstrates a postural-kinetic tremor from lesions of the cerebellar outflow pathways). Picking up small objects and performing fine movements will be impossible in the face of choreoathetosis and dyskinetic movement disorders. The simultaneous play of agonists and antagonists, the overflow of movement from adjacent muscle groups destroys pyramidal function. The examiner notes the influence of voluntary movement on the affected extremity. The only movement disorders that persist through sleep are Huntington's chorea and the dystonia of CRPS.

Epilepsy and convulsive movements

Partial motor seizures

Most major motor seizures are generalized from partial seizures. Seizures start by the synchronous firing of neurons in the cortex (the exception being the thalamus in petit mal seizures). This event is called a paroxysmal depolarization shift. The likelihood of a seizure occurring in a region of the cortex is determined by the afferent–efferent connections of the area, its collateral wiring characteristics and the ease of its depolarization. The most seizurogenic part of the brain is the medial temporal cortex. The primary motor and sensory cortex is next because of rich efferent and afferent connections with the reticular nuclei of the thalamus. It is less likely for a patient to experience a seizure from lesions of the far frontal, occipital and parietal lobes.

The representation of a body part on the sensory and motor homunculus and the ease with which these neurons depolarize determine the likelihood of that part of the brain firing from a cortical lesion.

A partial motor lesion of the lower portion of the motor homunculus starts with twitching of the thumb and fingers which quickly spreads to the corner of the mouth, the arm (skips the shoulders), the distal foot and then the entire rest of the body on that side. This is called a Jacksonian march. There is a large representation of the eyes in area 8 of the frontal cortex (frontal eye fields), the stimulation of which causes the head and eyes to deviate contralaterally with horizontal jerk nystagmus to the contralateral side of a seizure focus. If the Jacksonian march does not remit, the rest of the brain (seizures spread to the basal ganglia, substantia nigra, reticular nucleus of the thalamus and then cerebellum) will be recruited and it will generalize. A partial seizure usually lasts from 30–40 seconds to 2 minutes.

A generalized seizure usually starts abruptly with loss of consciousness and then rigidity of the arms and legs, and the head and eyes may deviate to either side. This represents the tonic phase of the seizure and corresponds to thalamic projections bilaterally to the motor cortex. This rigidity lasts for 15–20 seconds and is followed by the clonic phase, which consists of jerking of the face, neck, arms and legs. This process is inhibited by intra-cortical GABAergic inhibition from cortical interneurons and volleys from the cerebellum (the clonic phase), which is followed by another tonic discharge from reticular neurons of the thalamus. An epileptic cry at the onset of a generalized seizure is the expulsion of air through a partially opened larynx. Patients become cyanotic during a major motor seizure, they have excess saliva, tongue biting of the lateral tongue and urinary incontinence. A major motor seizure stops slowly with fewer and fewer jerking movements, which is followed by hyperhidrosis and stertorous breathing. Most major motor seizures last between 30 and 90 seconds. Post-ictal sleep may last for 20–30 minutes to hours. The side opposite the bitten tongue may be the hemisphere of origin of the seizure. The tip of the tongue is most often bitten with pseudoseizures. Some major motor seizures are only clonic while others just manifest the tonic phase. If a major motor seizure is bilateral, there is expected loss of consciousness (resulting from inhibition of the reticular thalamic nuclei).

Partial epilepsy may affect an extremity, the face or an entire side of the body without loss of consciousness. It may last for hours to days (Menshikoff's syndrome) and in older patients is most often caused by a vascular lesion, while in children it is Rasmussen's encephalitis. The syndrome is epilepsia partialis continua.

Seizures emanating from the supplementary motor cortex may display a speech arrest associated with contralateral dystonia, extensor posturing of the arm while the patient turns the head to the ipsilateral (seizure focus) with a flexed arm (fencer's posture).

Partial complex seizures emanating from the temporal lobe are associated with a variety of movements. If the patient suffers an automatism he or she will lose awareness, but continue his or her former activity or start a new stereotyped movement. Automatisms in general have three major components:

1   an arrest response in which the patient stops or slows motor activity;
2   an autonomic phase in which the patient is pale and has an expression-less face;
3   the movement phase.

A characteristic of the movement phase is lip smacking or chewing movements followed by stereotypical hand movements. A fugue state lasts for approximately 30 minutes to hours, in which a patient carries out normal activities, but has impairment of consciousness. Some partial seizures of temporal lobe origin are associated with contralateral dystonic arm posturing.

Typical absence seizures (petit mal seizures)

Many absence seizures have no motor manifestation. They consist of frequent episodes of loss of awareness that may be accompanied by twitching of the eyelids, dropping of the head, slight jerking of the hands and, rarely, repetitive speech. They may occur several hundred times a day and are eas-ily initiated by cerebral vasoconstriction induced by hyperventilation.

Myoclonic jerks

These are asymmetric movements primarily of the flexors of the upper extremities and extensors of the legs. In general, they move a joint and at times may be violent. The movements are sudden and often repetitive. In corticoreticular myoclonus (absence of cerebral cortical GABAergic inhibi-tion), they can be initiated by sound, touch or a loud noise. Myoclonic jerks are normal as a patient falls asleep. They usually affect the legs most severely and may spread to all extremities and disrupt sleep. These occur as part of the parasomniac movement complex and may accompany paroxys-mal REM sleep behavior disorders.

Myoclonic epilepsy of Janz usually starts in adolescence, affects the arms and is most pronounced after awakening or shortly thereafter. This form of seizure disorder may generalize to a motor seizure or remain as the only epileptic feature. Triggers may be eye closure, hyperventilation or sounds. Reticular myoclonus affects the cells of the nucleus gigantocellu-laris of the brainstem and is associated with metabolic abnormalities such as uremia, any hyperosmotic state or poisonings.

Segmental myoclonus is of spinal origin and used to be very common following the use of metrizamide contrast for myelography. It may be seen in metabolic abnormalities, most often hyperosmotic states (non-ketotic diabetic coma) or following spinal segmental arteriography.

Most corticoreticular myoclonus is from diffuse cortical degenerations that are associated with storage diseases of childhood and adolescence, Creutzfeldt–Jakob disease, advanced Alzheimer's and diffuse Lewy body disease as well as anoxic states. The Lance–Adams syndrome is an example of the latter in which a patient recovers from anoxia but has damaged sero-tonergic cells of the dorsal raphe of the thalamus. Myoclonic jerks are dram-atic with intentional movement in this syndrome.

Opisthotonus

Patients have extreme hyperactivity of extensor neurons of the spinal cord with opisthotonus. In its most extreme form, only the heels and back of the head may touch the bed. In tetanus (usually associated now with intravenous drug abuse) it is exacerbated by noise, emotion or touch. Maintained opisthotonus occurs with meningeal irritation in children or with severe extrapyramidal rigidity (Dawson's encephalitis in the Middle East – which is now very rare in the West). Intermittent decerebrate rigidity with adducted and internally rotated arms, extended feet that cannot be flexed is most often seen with transtentorial herniation from any source. Common examples are:

1 basal ganglionic or pontine hemorrhage;
2 severe head trauma;
3 brain tumor;
4 malignant intracerebral edema from middle cerebral artery stroke.

It is often provoked during tracheal irrigation in these severely ill, intubated patients.

Chorea

Chorea refers to quick movements of the extremities, no two of which are the same, which are often described as semipurposeful. They are associated with irregular respiration, rapid protrusion and retraction of the tongue (lizard-like) with a peculiar flapping of the tip. Volitional movements are exaggerated and choreatic eye movements show the same disorganized pattern of movement as do the extremities. In general, the patients are hypotonic but have normal or hyperactive reflexes. The small joints of the hand are hyperextended and bizarre postures of the fingers, toes and wrist are noted. The patient is unable to hold the arms and hands palm forward above the head, because the hands start to pronate. The tongue cannot be held out of the mouth. Movements lessen in repose. Patients rarely injure themselves but often drop objects. All forms of chorea have similar movements. These include:
1 Sydenham's chorea associated with emotional lability;
2 Huntington's chorea associated with severe dementia, choreatic eye movements and a lurching gait;
3 chorea of pregnancy (often the first) and that associated with oral contraceptive pills;
4 hereditary choreas;
5 chorea associated with polycythemia and anoxia.

Athetosis

This is a slow writhing movement of the trunk, wrist, fingers and ankles. The fingers writhe with a flexed wrist. There is slow adduction and outward abduction. The foot is plantar flexed and inverted. Athetosis ceases during sleep, is not affected by eye closure and is increased by voluntary movement. Respiration is normal, there is no tongue flap, but facial grimacing is prominent particularly with bilateral disease. There is a sinuous quality to the movements.

Athetosis is most often seen with anoxic birth injury, prenatal or perinatal strokes and with hemiparkinsonism. It is a feature of many heredofamilial syndromes and choreoathetosis. The combinations of chorea and athetosis is more commonly seen than either alone. The movements have a writhing sinuous component as well as the quick jerky movements of chorea. Abnormalities of wrist and finger posture as well as distal leg position are present. Either basic component of the process may predominate.

Respiratory rhythm and tongue movements are affected. The movements are exacerbated with voluntary effort and reinforcement (hand opening and closing) with one extremity exacerbating the involuntary movements of the other extremities.

Ataxia telangiectasia, syndromes associated with acanthocytosis (particularly neuroacanthocytosis), multiple heredofamilial syndromes associated with cognitive impairment as well as anoxic birth injury are causative.

Dyskinesias

This refers to all of the abnormal movements noted above. The disorder is now noted most frequently in late-stage Parkinson's disease with "peak dose dyskinesia" in combination with "wearing off akinesia." It may be most notable in the shoulders associated with athetosis. The choreic component is less rapid than in other choreas and the athetosis has smaller amplitude. Most patients with this disorder are now being treated with deep brain stimulation of the subthalamic nuclei with good success. At times, oral facial movements may be the most prominent.

Hemiballismus

Most patients with hemiballismus have suffered an embolic or thrombotic infarction of the subthalamic nucleus. The disorder is most common in diabetic and hypertensive patients. The interpeduncular artery from the top of the basilar (embolic pathology) or the thalamoperforate artery from the P1 segment of the posterior cerebral artery is most frequently affected. Patients present with a wildly flailing arm or leg. The proximal portions of the extremities are most frequently affected. The extremity demonstrates either constant movements or has intermittent episodes with short periods of repose.

Patients often restrain their upper extremity in their belt or under the contralateral arm. This disorder is not affected by eye closure, ceases with sleep and may be accompanied by increased tone and reflexes. Approximately two-thirds of the nucleus has to be infarcted to produce the movement. It is exhausting and interferes with nutrition and sleep. Patients may demonstrate an athetotic component particularly in the lower extremity. It almost always is of vascular origin, but has been seen with tumors and head injury.

Idiopathic generalized torsion dystonia

Seven major genetic forms of generalized dystonia have recently been described. Dystonia is an involuntarily held abnormal posture. The exact cerebral location is not known, but lesions of the putamen and motor thalamus have been documented. Peripheral and generalized dystonia is commonly seen in CRPS. In the hereditary forms, patients often present with a plantar flexed inverted foot. In peripheral dystonia from CRPS I or II (clear nerve injury in type II), the lower extremity is also plantar flexed and inverted while the upper extremity is flexed. In the severe genetic forms, the trunk and extremities demonstrate wide amplitude writhing movements, severe proximal joint movements with superimposed quicker smaller movements. Hypertrophy occurs in the affected muscles. This is frequently very marked in the sternocleidomastoid muscles if the process involves the head and neck.

Truncal athetoid movements

Athetoid movements comprise contractions of paraspinal and trunk muscles that cause arching of the back and lateral twisting of the torso associated with extreme rotation of the head and neck which last for 5–10 seconds. More rapid movements are seen at the initiation and end of the writhing movement. There is associated grimacing and protrusion of the tongue. Anxiety increases the movements and they are relieved by sleep and relaxation. Abnormal movements supervene when the patient attempts voluntary movement. The peripheral dystonias, particularly that seen with severe CRPS I or II, are not associated with this type of movement, but lock a patient in a flexed posture.

Involuntary movements of the face and neck

Facial tics

Tics are stereotypic repetitive movements that are usually unconscious and include blinking, pursing the lips, contraction on one side of the face or grimacing. They are exacerbated by anxiety, may be suppressed by concentration, often persist through adult life and are frequently associated with other patterned movements or vocalization. Patients may suppress the abnormal movement for a period of time, but an internal tension or desire to complete the movement (akathisia) becomes overwhelming and the tic ensures. The feeling of inner tension subsides as the movement is completed. The cycle of inner tension returns and the process is repeated. The associated movements often involve the shoulder girdle (abduction and forward rotation), retraction of the neck, contraction of the platysma and pectoral muscles. Rarely, an individual muscle may be affected.

Tics or habit spasms are common in childhood and decrease with adolescence. They are a major feature of Gilles de la Tourette syndrome, attentional deficit disorders, neuroacanthocytosis and Meige's syndrome. The latter affects the eyelids and mouth with excessive blinking and masseter movements. Tourette's is often associated with coughing, a clearing of the throat, a barking sound or compulsive swearing. There is accumulating evidence that these syndromes are associated with anatomic defects in the putamen, caudate and globus pallidus of the basal ganglia.

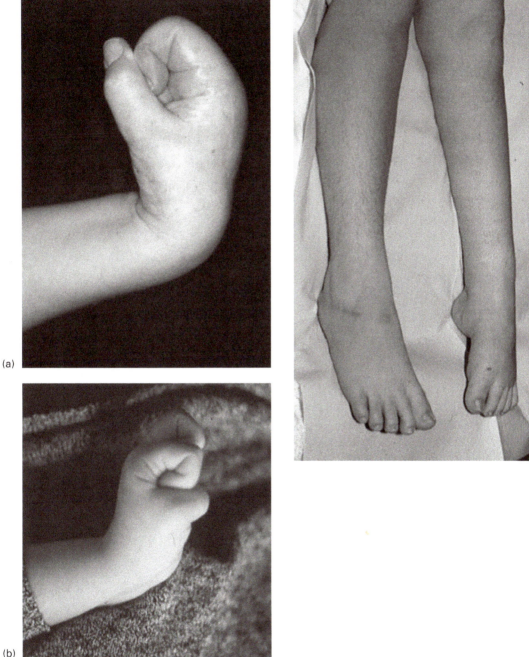

Fig. 6.1 Dystonia of chronic regional pain syndrome (CRPS). (a,b) Most dystonias of CRPS I and II are in flexion. They persist during sleep and are often accompanied by pain, neurogenic edema and dystrophy. (c) Characteristic plantar flexed and inverted foot dystonia of CRPS I and II.

Hemifacial spasms

Specific facial muscles spasmodically contract which usually contorts the face. The spasm starts with a few twitches of the orbicularis oculi and then spreads to specific facial muscles. Each spasm starts and stops suddenly, is increased by anxiety, suppressed at times by concentration or sleep and is stereotyped. Most of the time the spasm is caused by an aberrant loop of the anterior inferior cerebellar artery (AICA) that impinges upon the nerve and may be cured by the Jannetta procedure (removal of the artery from the nerve). Hemifacial spasm has also been described in tumors of the cerebellar pontine angle or aneurysms of AICA.

Aberrant regeneration of the seventh nerve (Bell's palsy) may cause a similar picture. However, the formerly denervated facial muscles are contracted (deep and prominent nasolabial fold), the spasm is initiated by voluntary movement and is often particularly prominent in the mentalis muscle. Fasciculations at rest may be observed.

Facial seizures may simulate facial palsy, but most frequently affect the eye or corner of the mouth, are slower and coarser, and stop by a gradual decrease of twitches. They are often accompanied by twitching of the thumb and hand.

Facial myokymia

These are undulating fine movements that are caused by firing of the terminal twigs of the facial nerve. In general, these flickering undulating movements are unilateral, but they may be bilateral. They have recently have been associated with autoimmune manifestations of an underlying cancer (antibodies to a K^+ channel), multiple sclerosis, vascular lesions of the pons and a few genetic conditions. Periorbital myokymia is benign, is restricted to the orbicularis oculi muscles, does not spread to the face and is seen with fatigue, lack of sleep and excess caffeine.

Perioral tremor

These are a group of peculiar mouthing movements often seen with the use of phenothiazine-based drugs. A constant coarse tremor of the orbicularis oris has been described with tertiary syphilis. A trombone protrusion of the tongue may be associated (protrusion and retraction) with this entity.

Spasmodic torticollis

This is forced turning of the head to the side, or rarely backwards (retrocollis). The chin is elevated and the occiput rotated and depressed. The spasms may be sustained, may occur as a rapid series with a normal interval and are often accompanied by overflow contractions of the platysma and facial muscles. They may be painful and frequently lead to cervical spondylosis that generates cracking sounds. They are increased by anxiety and lessened with relaxation. The sternocleidomastoid, scalene and strap muscles hypertrophy. It may be segmental or a component of generalized dystonia. Rarely, there is an aberrant artery unilaterally compressing the XI nerve. Fixed dystonia may be seen from cervical plexus (C1–C4 ventral root involvement which contribute to the innervation of the sternocleidomastoid (SCM) and scalene muscles) lesions often associated with the movement disorder of CRPS.

Facial dystonia and tardive dyskinesia

Bizarre grimacing, intermittent protrusion of a hypertrophied tongue most often occurs in concert with other features in a generalized dystonia. It may occur in isolation in Huntington's disease and Gilles de la Tourette syndrome, or as a major feature of some postanoxic states. Severe blepharospasm, occasionally to the point of interfering with vision, in combination with oromandibular dystonia is Meige's or Brueghel's syndrome. Meige's syndrome usually occurs in middle age and may be associated with spasmodic torticollis. These movements are more sustained and spasmodic in onset than those of tardive dyskinesia.

Tardive dyskinesia is characterized by a variety of peculiar mouthing or lip movements. They may start as uncontrollable movements of the tongue and quivering of the lips that are often stereotypical. They are occasionally associated with abnormal movements of the shoulder or hip girdle. Dyskinesia of the face may be prominent with excess D2 receptor stimulation of the face representation in the putamen during treatment of Parkinson's disease.

Titubation

This a vertical oscillation of the head noted in the upright position that disappears with recumbency. It is most often seen in demyelinating disease that destroys cerebellar connections. It is frequently associated with vermian posture (a flexed back) and side-to-side swaying. Essential tremor causes a side-to-side head tremor. A "bobble head" tremor, which is a nonstereotypical vertical head tremor, is noted with third ventricular tumors. Rarely, a vertical head tremor is seen in severe Parkinson's disease. Isolated head nodding is noted in early torticollis.

Tremors (Fig. 6.2)

Tremors are symmetric movements of a body part. There are central generators in the thalamus and cerebellum whose discharge sets the frequency of the tremor. Peripheral feedback from proprioceptive joint fibers that are moved exacerbate or inhibit tremors. Abnormalities of proprioceptive and other somatic fibers from peripheral nerves may initiate and sustain

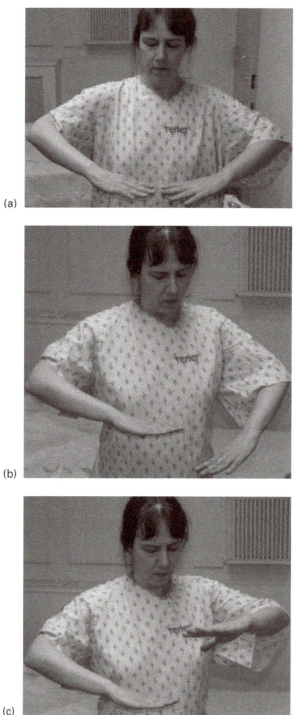

(a)

(b)

(c)

Fig. 6.2 (a) Postural kinetic tremor. Patient attempts to maintain her arms in a sustained posture. (b) Downward oscillation of the left arm and hand. (c) Upward oscillation of the left arm and hand. The greater the oscillation, the closer the lesion is to the red nucleus. A lesion has interrupted the dentatorubral thalamic pathway.

tremors. A fine tremor is difficult to see. It can be amplified if it is in the upper extremity by placing a piece of paper on the outstretched fingers. A coarse tremor most often is slower than a fine tremor, but only moves the extremity a few millimeters. There are several non-specific triggers for tremors. A postural-kinetic tremor occurs when the patient tries to maintain a fixed posture. There is a postural tremor that occurs only when the patient is in the upright posture (orthostatic tremor). Central axial and

146

head tremor may be more prominent than appendicular or extremity tremors in this entity. Tremors associated with basal ganglia disease are noted at rest. They are invariably associated with abnormalities of posture and flexed metacarpophalangeal joints of the hand.

Nervousness

This is the most common tremor that is universal and physiologic. It affects the hands most prominently, although when severe the voice, body and extremities may be involved. It is present at rest and increased with voluntary movement and is not increased by automatic movements. This tremor is physiologic resulting from β-adrenergic stimulation of the segmental stretch reflex and is between 10 and 15 Hz.

The anxiety state

This is similar to that caused by nervousness and is caused by excess circulating noradrenaline from the periphery of the adrenal gland as well as that released from discharge of sympathetic neurons of the intermediolateral column of the spinal cord. It is coarser than a physiologic tremor and is associated with dilated pupils, tachycardia, hyperhidrosis, and cold and sweaty hands.

Thyrotoxicosis

This is a persistent rapid tremor most clearly demonstrated in the extremities by resting a piece of paper on the outstretched limbs. It is accompanied by pathologic lid retraction (Collier's sign), tachycardia and hyperhidrosis with warm extremities. The circulation is hyperdynamic, venous pulsations on the optic disk are exaggerated and it responds to β-adrenergic blocking agents.

Alcoholism

The ataxia of alcoholism affects the legs more than the arms; there is a "martinette" gait and patients have minimal nystagmus. The tremor is postural, between 6 and 11 Hz, is present constantly and is minimally influenced by emotion or voluntary movement. It may be associated with Quinquaud's sign. The examiner presses his or her palms against the patient's outstretched fingertips and there is flexion of the metacarpophalangeal joints and extension of the distal interphalangeal joints. The proximal joints of the extremity are not fixed in proper position to allow a solid base for pyramidal movements. This tremor and these signs are caused by cerebellar dysfunction which regulates agonist and antagonist muscle control at proximal and distal joints. The tremor of acute alcohol withdrawal may be close to 8 Hz which is similar to essential tremor.

Toxic tremors

Withdrawals from opiates cause an enhanced physiologic tremor resulting from sympathetic nervous system stimulation. Lithium causes a wide variety of abnormal movements including myoclonus, postural kinetic tremor and a coarse tremor of the outstretched extremities. Lithium and nicotine can both mimic an alcohol-type tremor. Toluene abuse, along with other solvents, may produce a severe intention tremor.

Essential tremor

This may be seen in two major varieties. There are both autosomal dominant (AD) and autosomal recessive (AR) forms, with variable penetrance and interfamilial and intrafamilial variance. Some have a more marked rapid side-to-side head tremor with less difficulty with intention while others have a coarser side-to-side head tremor and slower intention tremor. The tremor is constant and worsened by emotional upset and decreased by alcohol (approximately 20 minutes after one glass of white wine). The tremor will stop at the instant of execution of a fine movement (marked while holding the arms outstretched, but absent on picking up a pencil). This particular component of the tremor is noted as a postural action tremor. The tremor can be purely intentional and its usual frequency is 8 Hz.

Parkinsonian tremor

This is a characteristic pill-rolling tremor. The hand is flexed at the metacarpophalangeal joint and there is a flexion–extension movement of the thumb. As the tremor progresses in severity, the thumb rubs against the forefinger which initiates a flexion tremor at the first interphalangeal joint. Further progression of the tremor causes all fingers of the hand to flex together. It is exacerbated by emotion and is present at rest. The tremor is absent with total relaxation, during sleep and immediately after awakening. It is suppressed by initiation of voluntary movements. In severe patients it persists through voluntary movement and has postural kinetic components (maintaining a proximal joint posture). It is associated with a forward flexed posture, the other manifestations of Parkinson's disease and, most importantly, cog-wheel rigidity of the wrist and fingers. The head tremor is up and down, but is rare. There is an association with essential tremor (higher incidence of essential tremor in first-degree relatives). In severe Parkinson's disease, tremor is rarely extreme as most patients are taking levodopa therapy or have had deep brain stimulation that is effective. The akinetic-rigid states such as FTD-17 dementia, MSA and corticobasal ganglia degeneration have no tremor. Tremor is not a feature of drug-induced parkinsonism.

Tremor in collagen disease

Chorea is characteristic of systemic lupus erythematosus (SLE). A coarse, side-to-side, irregular tremor of the digits (finger playing similar to polyminimyoclonus) has been described particularly in periarteritis nodosa. It is increased by postural maintenance, emotional upset and disappears with total relaxation.

Intention tremor

This is a coarse tremor (4–6 Hz) that is absent at rest and occurs during the last one-third of a voluntary movement. The last third of a voluntary movement is then affected by side-to-side oscillation as the target is approached. It may be extremely severe which precludes effective voluntary movement. In the milder forms it can be enhanced by having the patient hold the finger gently on the tip of the nose. This reflects a lesion of the cerebellum or its connections. The most common pathology is multiple sclerosis, but it is clearly noted in cerebellar infarction, usually of AICA or the spinocerebella atrophy (SCA), postanoxic states or genetic cerebellar disease.

Red nucleus tremor (rubral tremor) (see Fig. 6.2)

This tremor is most often caused by a vascular lesion of the thalamoperforate artery from the posterior cerebral or paramedian arteries whose origin is the top of the basilar artery (usually embolic). The tremor is unilateral, slow coarse and rhythmic (Claude's syndrome). It is present at rest (minimally) and throughout all components of a voluntary movement. It is at a right angle to the line of movement and is often concomitant with ataxia. The lesion interrupts dentate cerebellar outflow afferents as they pass near the red nucleus ("en passage") to the thalamus. It is claimed that the closer the lesion is to the red nucleus the more marked and worse the tremor will be. It is often accompanied by a contralateral third nerve palsy and there are choreoathetoid movements of the contralateral extremities (Benedict's syndrome). A rubral tremor is 2.5–4.0 Hz in frequency and increases in amplitude as the hand reaches the target. There is a concomitant postural kinetic component of the affected arm. The tremor has been well described in demyelinating disease and following severe closed head injury.

Tremor in Wilson's disease

This is a vertical, asymmetric, irregular flapping tremor that involves the wrist and shoulder girdle. It is increased by voluntary movement and has choreic and intention components. It is absent in repose, but is immediately evident when the patient attempts to fix the limb or maintain a specific posture (postural kinetic). A Kayser–Fleischer ring (golden crescent in the superior part of the iris in a blue-eyed patient) is pathognomonic. Patients are extremely dysarthric, demented, hypotonic and hyperreflexic.

"The wing flap"

This is described as a wing-flapping tremor of the wrists noted as a precursor to hepatic coma.

Asterixis

This is a sudden loss of extensor postural tone. The patient is asked to hold the arms outstretched with the wrists dorsiflexed. There is a sudden loss of tone, the wrist drops and then there is a compensatory jerk to reposition the hand to its former position. It is seen in hepatic, pulmonary and renal failure as well as hyperosmotic states and poisoning. It is particularly helpful in the unconscious state as it suggests a metabolic etiology. It is a form of negative myoclonus.

Pseudoathetosis or "sensory wandering" in association with updrifts (Fig. 6.3)

These movements are caused by severe proprioceptive loss. Most commonly, this is of peripheral origin from destruction of large dorsal root

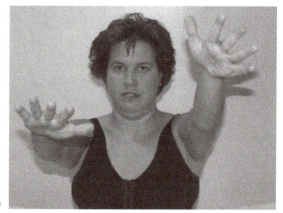

(a)

(b)

Fig. 6.3 Finger wandering/updrifts. Finger-playing movement of the hand without proprioception. Often injury to the dorsal root ganglia. (a) Parietal updrift. The hand drifts up and out, with or without sinuous movements of the finger. (b) Thalamic updrift. The wrist flexes with the thumb adducting into the middle palm.

ganglia neurons (autoimmune or toxic etiology), a large fiber peripheral neuropathy or a central lesion of the lemniscal pathways. It is most easily demonstrated by having the patient hold the arms outstretched or placing the extremity on a flat surface. Sinuous wandering movements of the fingers are seen that are accompanied by wrist flexion at the metacarpophalangeal joints which will elevate the extremity from a flat surface. The fingers close, the wrist further flexes and the arm is internally rotated. The movements are suppressed if the patient watches the hand, which cannot be done with athetosis. There is always associated loss of large fiber mediated position sense. Similar involuntary movements are noted in the lower extremities. In tabes dorsalis the large proprioceptive fibers of the dorsal root entry zone ganglia and the dorsal columns are affected and this constituted "tabetic athetosis." It is noted with severe degeneration of the dorsal columns that occurs with degenerative disease, HIV, myelopathy, autoimmune or carcinomatous large fiber destruction, Sjögren's disease and vitamin B$_{12}$ deficiency.

Dramatic proprioceptive loss occurs with dorsal column nuclear lesions. Movements attempted in this condition produce wide oscillations and a lateral drift of the outstretched upper extremities.

Parietal lesions cause an updrift of the extremity contralateral to the lesion that has angular displacement of the hand with finger-playing sinuous movements (see Fig. 6.3a). A similar updrift occurs with thalamic lesions of the major sensory nucleus ventroposterior lateral (VPL), but is distinguished from a parietal lesion by flexion of the wrist and adduction of the thumb into the palm (see Fig. 6.3b).

Movements limited to muscles

Fasciculation

This is a movement caused by abnormal firing of an entire motor unit (the anterior horn cell, the axons, the terminal, twigs and the individual sarcolemmal fibers). The closer the lesion is to the anterior horn cell the more fasciculations are noted. The movements are irregular, non-rhythmic contractions of the muscle unit caused by spontaneous firing of anterior horn cells or their axons. The movements do not displace a joint, are coarse or fine, and are most easily seen in the deltoid, quadriceps and calves although they can occur in any muscle group. They are present at rest and suppressed with voluntary movement, but are exacerbated afterwards.

They are facilitated by heat or provoked by mechanically stimulating the muscle (striking it with a percussion hammer). They usually are not felt by the patient unless they are dramatic and fire large muscle units as occurs in ALS. If significant, there is associated weakness and atrophy of the affected muscle. The anterior or ventral roots are often affected in severe cervical spondylosis which causes fasciculation and atrophy of the deltoid, biceps and triceps muscles.

Fibrillations are fine movements of sarcomeres (one muscle fiber). They can most easily be seen in the tongue because there is no overlying sub-cutaneous tissue. In motor neuron disease (ALS), peripheral atrophy, a hyperactive jaw jerk and increased extremity reflexes are also seen. In syringobulbia, fibrillation of the tongue with associated atrophy occurs, but there is a normal jaw jerk. Fasciculations of the calves occur with radiculopathies affecting the S1 root, arachnoiditis, old polio, syphilitic amyotrophy and as a benign condition. The cramp fasciculation syndrome causes fasciculations and cramps in exercised muscle without weakness or atrophy. After, discharges are noted in the affected muscles. Thyrotoxicosis may demonstrate particular wasting of the rhomboids, weakness of the iliopsoas and have fasciculations with absent reflexes. Fibrillations of the tongue have been described with hyperparathyroidism and hyperthyroid-ism without associated weakness and wasting. Rarely, Kennedy's syndrome, a trinucleotide CAG repeat disease, affects the pharynx and tongue along with striking fasciculations of the face. There is associated gynecomastia (from a mutation that affects the androgen receptor).

Clonus

This is a rapid extension flexion movement of a group of muscles that is regular, occurs in association with a hypertonic limb which is hyperreflexic. It is triggered most often by a rapid displacement of the limb that increases its tone (dorsiflexion of the ankle). It can be stopped by decreasing the tone of the muscle.

7: Basic Principles for the Sensory Examination

This is the most difficult and least objective part of the neurologic examination because a major portion of it is under the control of the patient. However, the good examiner is armed with an understanding of the innervation patterns of the body surface which are root, nerve or false radiations (somatic visceral convergence) or are central patterns of deficits that are reflected on the body surface. The nerve bundles themselves have nervi-nervorum which, if sensitized, cause pain when the bundle is compressed. Frequently in radiculopathy, the muscle that receives innervation is sore on mechanical compression (sensitization) because nociceptive afferents which usually do not respond to simple pressure do so when they are sensitized. Thus, a disk that compresses the S1 root which carries deep muscle pain afferents (A-delta fibers) causes the gastrocnemius muscle to hurt when compressed. This occurs because these A-delta receptors, which normally only respond to tissue destructive stimuli, are now sensitized and respond to mechanical stimuli. Similarly, the same disk at S1 may sensitize the roots (L4–S2) in the sciatic notch so that when it is compressed the patient feels pain at the notch, but not in other areas of the sciatic nerve innervation. Use of the thumb by the examiner on sensitized muscles and nerves, confirmed with careful observations of the patient, objectifies much of the sensory examination. Knowledge of the entrance points of the nerves through the thoracic inlet and outlet, the neurovascular bundle (medial to the humerus) and then the tunnels into the forearm (cubital, arcade of Frohse and the pronator canal) allow the examiner to palpate and judge the sensitivity of the nerves. Placing the plexus in specific positions (Roos' abduction stretch maneuver, Wright's maneuver) places different components of the plexus under traction and spontaneously fire. Compression of the cervical roots as they exit the cervical foramina (Spurling's maneuver) allows identification of specific nerve root irritation.

There is now a great deal of molecular biologic information that explains the mechanisms in which chronic afferent painful stimuli change the physiology of the spinal cord. This phenomena causes mechano- and thermal allodynia such that an innocuous stimulus causes pain. Similarly, in hyperalgesia, a normally painful stimulus is perceived as too painful. The most extreme manifestation of abnormal spinal cord processing of painful stimuli occurs with hyperpathia. In this condition, which may be caused by peripheral nerve root or fiber damage as well as central lesions of pain pathways, there is:

1   a higher threshold to perceive pain;
2   an abnormally rapid increase of pain to maximal intensity;
3   that is overwhelming in intensity;
4   is not stimulus bound.

Patterns of sensory loss from central lesions are often diagnostic and will be illustrated and described below.

Modalities of sensation to be tested

Each sensory modality has a specific receptor in the skin, muscle, joint and bone. Each type of receptors information is relayed to the spinal cord by a specific-sized neuron whose cell body is in the dorsal root ganglia and has a peripheral projection to the innervated areas as well as to the gray matter of the spinal cord. The transmitters for pain glutamate and aspartate are localized both in the peripheral nerve endings and centrally in the dorsal horn concomitantly with neuropeptides such as substance P and calcitonin gene-related peptide (CGRP). This is important new information because it helps explain some associated features of peripheral nerve, root and "C" and A-delta fiber damage.

Each modality of sensation is carried by a specific fiber size. Thus, the type of sensory perception felt by the patient identifies the size of the fiber affected or its central projections. This is extremity valuable in localization of the sensory deficit. There is a great deal of sensory processing at all levels which modifies sensory stimuli.

Modalities of sensation that are tested at the bedside

1   Pain, light touch and temperature. Pain is usually tested with a pin, while light touch can be evaluated with the hand or a wisp of cotton. The tuning fork is used both for vibration sensibility and to test cold. Burning pain is carried by "C" (1 μm) fibers. A-delta fibers are 1–4 μm and carry lancinating pain (that which occurs with root disease), sharp pain and cold. Heat is carried by another subgroup of polymodal C fibers. The sensation of light touch is mediated by A-B fibers which are 8–10 μm in diameter. They also mediate tap, some deep muscle pressure and dynamic allodynia (lightly stroking of the skin that is painful). This pain is associated with central sensitization and occurs in chronic regional pain syndrome (CRPS), some central pain states and in the dermatomes adjacent to those affected by herpes zoster.

2   Position sense is mediated by large A-alpha fibers that innervate muscle, joints and tendons and also mediate vibration sensibility. These are the largest axons and are 12–22 μm in diameter. They mediate the paresthetic sense of tingling. A loss of proprioceptive input from central lesions is often reported as sense of numbness or heaviness. Sympathetic fibers do not carry sensation, but may drive and increase the firing rate of central pain projecting neurons in the central nervous system and exacerbate many pain states.

3 Stereognosis, two-point discrimination, graphesthesias, the ability to copy posture and to record two simultaneous stimuli are elaborated sensations and derive from the primary afferent input. They are most frequently lost from cortical and thalamic lesions.

Essential features of the sensory pathways

A root lesion will cause loss of all sensation that it carries. There is a segregation of root fibers, the most lateral of those that enter the spinal cord carry pain and temperature. A protruded disk often herniates laterally and compresses this component of the dorsal root entry zone. The dorsal root ganglia are in the foraminal exit foramina of the spine. Lesions between the ganglia and the spinal cord most often cause lancinating pain (A-delta fibers are affected) while those from the dorsal root ganglia (DRG) to the periphery cause numbness.

Pain and temperature fibers are subserved by polymodal naked "C" fibers (unmyelinated) that innervate all tissues of the body. A-delta, 1-μm fibers are thinly myelinated and carry lancinating sharp pain and cold, while the "C" fibers carry slow and burning pain. A class of C fibers mediates itch.

Pain fibers may be thought of as mediating two major systems. The first are those that record the location and frequency of firing of the activated "C" and A-delta fibers and a second group that mediate the affect of pain and starts the process of pain behavior. The first group synapse on neurons in Rexed Layer I of the substantia gelatinosa of the dorsal horn and ascend through the brainstem to the ventral posterolateral nuclei of the thalamus and then to the primary sensory area of the cortex SI. There are multiple collaterals from these pain afferents which underlie pain mechanisms and behavior. As these pain afferents enter the dorsal horn they are distributed 1–2 segments above and below the segment they innervate by Lissauer's tract of the spinal cord. They have collaterals that synapse on the intermediolateral column neurons of the spinal cord (the origin of the sympathetics) as well as the anterior horn cells (motor neurons) of Rexed Layer IX. Thus, a painful stimulus activates and drives sympathetic fibers as well as motor fibers. A very painful injury will cause a complicated nocifensor response of flexor neurons that causes splinting and a sympathetic response that changes blood flow. The more severe the afferent painful barrage and the longer it is maintained, the innervated segments above and below the major segmental afferent input will fire and the patient will have pain or hypersensitivity of these adjacent spinal segments. This is the beginning of a process of central sensitization that underlies many chronic pain states. The status of the *N*-methyl-ᴅ-aspartate (NMDA) receptors both on pain afferents and on central pain projecting neurons (CPPN) of the dorsal horn of the spinal cord determines if sensitization occurs. The firing of one pain fiber and one central pain projecting neuron can be localized and recorded. The more the pain fiber discharges and the central pain projecting neuron fires the greater the severity of the pain. If the CPPN or the "C" fiber fires spontaneously, the patient suffers spontaneous pain.

There is another group of pain nociceptors that innervate Rexed Layer II of the substantia gelatinosa which mediates the affectual components of pain. These fibers project to the amygdala of the temporal lobe, brainstem nuclei, the anterior cingulate gyrus, SII of the cortex, posterior insular cortex and dorsolateral prefrontal cortex. This system is modulated by monoaminergic uptake blockers, narcotics and frontal lobectomies. This system determines pain behavior.

A third anatomic system that subserves pain is that mediated by wide dynamic neurons (WDR) of the dorsal horn in Rexed Layer V. These neurons receive inputs from low threshold afferents, sympathetic fibers and nociceptive specific fibers (which signal tissue destruction). Thus, at a spinal level there is convergence of sympathetic, touch and pain input on a group of neurons that if stimulated signal pain. The axons from these neurons cross below the central canal in conjunction with axons from Rexed Layers I and II to form the spinothalamic tract. This system has rich collaterals with brainstem nuclei, the periaqueductal gray of the midbrain, the lateral aspects of the reticular formation at all levels, the intralaminar nuclei of the thalamus and projects bilaterally to SI and SII of the cortex. The major components of this system are contralateral.

The sensation of pain of all sorts drives the patient to the physician. It must be understood that the system is dynamic and plastic. Molecular biology has entered this arena in a major way. In a dramatic oversimplification, chronic pain inputs turn on immediate early response genes both in the DRG (origin of pain fibers), which in turn activate translational factors that initiate transcription of the DNA of the DRG and Rexed Layer I, II and V cells, which then manufacture different sodium channels and new proteins that change the firing characteristics of the system. If it is up-regulated there is central sensitization, the clinical expression of which is allodynia, hyperalgesia and hyperpathia (also known as long-term potentiation (LTP) and if it is down-regulated the patient cannot appreciate pain (long-term depression (LTD)).

The spinothalamic tract is laminated so that sacral and lumbar fibers are most lateral within the pathway and the arm and hand are most medial. The fibers cross to the contralateral side at the segment they enter the cord. The spinothalamic tract is lateral and the lemniscal pathways (mediate vibration, proprioception and discreet touch) are medial throughout central pathways. Pain fibers from the face project to the fifth nucleus and then cross medially in the medulla and join spinothalamic fibers in the pons. Pain and touch sensations for the face can be dissociated at a pontine level. Facial fibers for touch synapse in the pons. A medullary midline lesion will cause a numb mid face because the quintospinothalmaic tract carrying pain crosses bilaterally in the midline. There are many variations of spinothalamic sensory loss that depend on the degree of damage to descending facial fibers that are ipsilateral (prior to crossing in the medulla in the quintothalamic tract) and the adjacent ascending spinothalamic tract (STT) that has crossed at its level of entry. Thus, a lateral medullary lesion that damages ipsilateral descending facial fibers will cause loss of ipsilateral pain and temperature sensation in the face and in the contralateral sacrum leg, trunk and arm distribution because of destruction of the STT that has crossed at its level of entry and ascends from the contralateral part of the body. The face is involved on the side of the lesion and there is loss of pinprick and cold contralaterally below the clavicle.

A lesion in the pons where the quintothalamic (facial fibers) and the extremity and body fibers have joined will cause total loss of pain and temperature contralaterally. A similar deficit will occur from a thalamic nuclear lesion that destroys the ventral posteromedial and posterolateral thalamic nuclei (VPM and VPL). In general, cortical lesions do not affect pain sensitivity to a great degree because it is bilaterally represented from SII and from bilateral projections of the intralaminar thalamic nuclei. The affective components of pain (the same as those affected from frontal lobotomies) may be affected from cortical lesions. Destruction of SII (at the foot of SI) has caused inability to appreciate pain.

Fibers carrying light touch, proprioception and vibration ascend in the posterior columns ipsilaterally to the nucleus gracilis and cuneatus, cross in the decussation slightly anterior to the pyramidal decussation at C1–C2 to join the medial lemniscus and project to VPL and VPM nuclear groups. Touch fibers from the face form part of this projection in the brainstem. The neospinothalamic pathways (anterior spinothalamic tract) enters the spinal cord, ascends and crosses to join the lateral spinothalamic tract. Central cord lesions affect pain and temperature (they decunate in the midline) but not light touch to a major degree as a result of this innervation. The lateral cervical nucleus is found at C1–C4 levels and relays both touch and proprioceptive information to the contralateral thalamus. This appears to be the fastest sensory pathway (from the ipsilateral arm) to the cortex and sets it for further sensory information.

Position and vibratory sensation fibers originate in the large cells of the DRG. These neurons may be surrounded by sympathetic fibers after peripheral nerve injury (baskets that are able to depolarize them). There is another peripheral source of sympathetic somatic interaction. Pain fibers that are abnormally active up-regulate their α-adrenoreceptors. Pain afferents are driven by sympathetic discharge that they initiate (collaterals from their afferent input) and are maintained by means of collaterals of that synapse on the neurons of the intermediolateral column of the dorsal horn. These are the connections that comprise the spinal somatosympathetic system. Once large afferents, 12–22 μm, that carry position, vibration and some light touch sensibility enter the cord, they ascend in the dorsal columns to synapse on the nucleus cuneatus (arm) and gracilis (leg) which form the medial lemniscus. It decussates slightly anterior to the decussation of the corticospinal pathways at C1–C2. They travel a medial course throughout the brainstem to synapse in the VPM and VPL. They also have a rich collateral network throughout their course and are joined by touch fibers from the face. Lesions of the dorsal column nuclei cause severe proprioceptive deficits, flailing gyrations of the arms during attempted voluntary movement and grave difficulty with walking. Thalamic lemniscal lesions are associated with a specific hand posture on drift testing and peculiar postures of the extremities in bed. The patient may be seen to lie on the arm that is twisted underneath. Parietal lesions are suspected when a patient has a large element of neglect and is lying at an angle in bed, ignoring the side opposite the lesion. Dorsal column nuclei and thalamic lesions are the only locations that cause loss of vibration sensibility. Neglect of external space may occur at any level of a sensory lesion, but is most severe at cortical levels. Recent anatomic information details a visceral pain pathway in the ventral components of the dorsal columns. The lateral cervical nucleus is located above the corticospinal pathways in the cervical spinal cord and also carries vibration and proprioceptive information to the thalamus and SI of the cortex. Sacral fibers are located dorsally in the posterior columns. In VPL, the leg trunk and arm are laminated laterally to medially. The face is represented in VPM. There is a newly described posterior inferior nucleus behind VPM/VPL that may be important for pain. The ventral thalamic posterior inferior (VPI) nucleus is a small thalamic nucleus inferior to VPL in which finger fibers are discrete. A small lesion here will cause numbness of the tips of all fingers. Pseudothalamic type sensory loss can occur from a lesion of the primary sensory cortex (SI) known as Vernet's syndrome. The leg area of SI is near the sagittal sinus. Representation of the genitalia is in the medial wall of the hemisphere and the trunk, arm and face are ventral in the postcentral gyrus. The face and hand representation are large with the thumb juxtaposed to the lip.

Sensory dermatomes (Fig. 7.1)

Roots overlap at least one segment above and one segment below their level of entry into the cord. Chronic neuropathic pain, which will be dealt with most by the neurologist and all practitioners, causes dynamic and plastic changes in pain systems that often cause painful states which have a regional rather than nerve or dermatomal pattern.

Throughout modern times, neurologists have not understood brachial and cervical plexus distributions which are frequently confused with root and nerve distributions. These will be dealt with in some detail because a great number of mistakes are made in this area.

Dermatomal charts present the patient standing with the palms forward:
1   C1: no somatic supply on the skin surface
2   C2: occiput and the angle of the jaw
3   C3: anterior neck
4   C4: trapezius ridge
5   C5: outer aspect of the shoulder tip
6   C6: lateral forearm, thumb and index finger (rare involvement)
7   C7: triceps; middle finger (rare involvement)

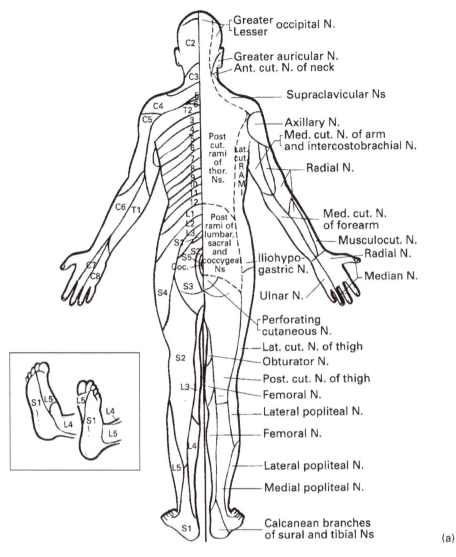

Fig. 7.1 (a,b) Outline of the sensory segmental dermatomes and average area of peripheral nerve supply. Individual variability is considerable. (*Cont'd on page 160*).

8 C8: fourth and fifth fingers

9 C8–T1: sympathetic fibers to the eye (superior cervical sympathetic ganglia)

10 T2: sympathetic supply to the arm (travels with the lower trunk of the brachial plexus)

11 T4: level of the nipple (also dropped sensory level from the cervical cord)

12 T6: tip of the scapula (notalgia from upper trunk of the brachial plexus)

13 T8: rib margin

14 T10: umbilicus

15 T12: pubis

16 L1: groin (also radiation of S1, this radiation is common)

17 L3: middle knee

18 L4: inner knee; medial leg; band sensation around the ankle

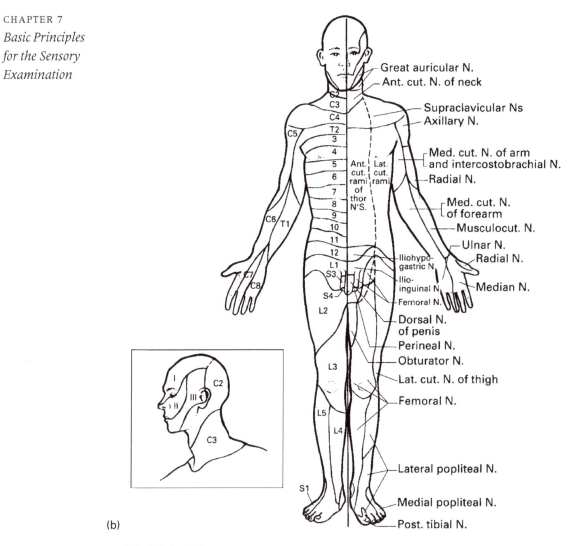

(b)

Fig. 7.1 *(cont'd)*

19 L5: lateral thigh; scrotum (projected radiation; anterior thigh-dural radiation of L5 – the recurrent nerve of Spurling); the lateral knee (part of the recurrent nerve of Gonyea, a branch of the posterior tibial nerve)

20 S1: lateral side of the bottom of the foot; small toe; projected radiation (tip of the penis, groin; inside the vagina unilaterally)

21 S3–S5: concentric rings around the anus; some patients seem to innervate the anus most medially with S1

As a general rule, cervical nerve roots do not project to the hand unless they are severely irritated. Nerves and brachial plexus lesions project to the hand. C8 and T1 are not motion segments. Rarely does anything happen at this level other than severe trauma or metastatic disease. C6–C7 most often projects down the midline of the spine. The brachial plexus upper trunk radiation is down the medial scapular border. C2 (dural radiation) is often to the brow. T1 is the inner side of the upper arm and C5 is the cap of the shoulder. Thus, within 2.5 cm on the surface of the arm is C5–T1. C8–T1 lesions are often accompanied by a Horner's syndrome.

The most important roots of the lower extremity are L5 and S1. This is the major motion segment and all forms of arthritis, disk and mechanical problems occur here. L5 has radiations into the hip, scrotum, posterior popliteal fossa, anterior leg to the big toe. It also projects to the under surface of the foot medially. The dural projection of L5 is to the anterior thigh (recurrent nerve of Spurling). This is always mistaken for L1–L3. S1 has a radiation to the groin that is always mistaken for L1. One side of the vagina can clearly be discerned from a unilateral lesion of S1. The most convincing radiations of S1 are to the little toe and the calf. The S1 root also projects to the sciatic notch, the sacroiliac joint and to the tip of the penis.

The major nerves that need to be learnt are the median, ulnar, radial, intercosticobrachial (derived from the medial cord of the brachial plexus), the sciatic peroneal, saphenous and plantar nerves. These will be illustrated in detail under patterns of sensory loss.

The patterns of sensory loss that are most often missed are those of the cervical and brachial plexus with their derivative peripheral nerves. The most common cause of atypical chest pain is the intercosticobrachial nerve that derives from the medial cord of the brachial plexus.

Pain, touch and temperature

Preliminary screening

It is helpful to start the sensory examination by explaining to the patient that he or she will not be punctured by the examiner's pin. Explain, "I am not going to hurt you," so relax. Touch the patient on a normal part of the body and ask what he or she feels. It should be a pricking sensation that is not painful. The pin is then used to determine the pattern of sensory deficit. If it is peripheral, the examiner should have determined if it is in a root nerve or plexus distribution. If a central lesion is suspected, the level of the lesion should be determined. Nothing in neurology happens in a vacuum. The history has already led the examiner to the correct type of problem. If the patient is a typist and has a numb hand, the examiner suspects carpal tunnel syndrome. The history has elucidated further that the patient is awakened at night by numbness in the hand, which is relieved by hanging the hand over the side of the bed. The examiner demonstrates a Tinel's sign (tapping over the carpal tunnel) which produces paresthesias into the thumb, index and long finger. The tip of the index finger is numb and the patient has more feeling in the lateral than medial portion of the fourth finger. If on the other hand, the patient has suffered the sudden onset of nausea and vomiting, falls to the side and has difficulty swallowing, the examiner expects a loss of sensation (pin prick and temperature) in the ipsilateral face and the contralateral side of the body below the clavicle: a brainstem posterior inferior cerebellar artery (PICA) vascular distribution.

As a general rule, it is better to examine from an area of impaired sensation to one of normal sensation, which is easier to detect by the patient. Ask if there is a difference between two areas and what the difference is.

Touch

The examiner uses a small cotton wisp. One can use the hand for light touch over the affected area. Pressure will stimulate deep afferents as well as A-delta and C-afferents that innervate muscle, tendon and periosteum if they are sensitized.

Temperature

Temperature and pain test small fibers. On the face, patients are more comfortable with temperature testing than with pinprick. The tuning fork may be used to test cold (mediated by A-delta thinly myelinated afferents). Rarely, in patients with neuropathies that affect warm "C" fiber endings in tissue, a test tube heated to 43°C may be used to test heat which is mediated by 1 μm C fibers. Rarely, there is transmodality modulation in the spinal cord where cold is perceived as heat. This may also occur at a receptor level in the skin. It is noted in ciguatera poisoning (fish from the Caribbean) as well as in CRPS I or II.

Sensory levels

Sensory levels on the trunk have several pitfalls. In general, at a dermatome level, the loss is 1–2 segments higher at the back than the front (the same tilt as the intercostal nerves). The lamination of the spinothalamic tract is such that the sacrum is represented laterally with leg, trunk and arm medially. Thus, a lateral lesion of the cord and may give a dropped level so that a cervical lesion on the right causes loss of pinprick in the left lower leg. The spinothalamic tract (STT) crosses and innervates above and below 1–2 segments from its level of entry into the cord. The posterior columns (lemniscal input) is laminated with the leg fibers medially and the arms represented more laterally. The sacrum is represented dorsally. A central cord lesion affects the arms and tends to spare sacral dermatomes. The spinal segments do not completely correlate with the named vertebrae at that segment. In C1–C6 they do, but at the C8 spinal segment the corresponding vertebra is C7. At upper thoracic levels, a lesion may cause a two spinal segments drop in level. The lumbar and sacral segments are opposite the T11–L1 vertebrae. In essence, the spinal cord is pulled up within the vertebral segments.

Spinal cord lesions should be tested both for an upper and lower level because of the lamination of the major sensory pathways which produces sacral sparing.

Remember that T3–T4 is close to C4 on the chest (infraclavicular nerve), T2–C5 are adjacent in the arm (T2 medial humerus, C5 cap of the shoulder) and S2–L2 in the thigh.

Objective sensory testing

Most sensory testing is dependent on the response of the patient. Testing proprioception in the extremities is under control of the examiner. A patient should be able to detect a 1° displacement of the distal phalanx in the upper extremity and 5° of displacement in the lower extremity. It is often good to ask the patient to tell which toe is being held (fourth vs fifth). Skin proprioception is also an objective way to quantify a sensory level. Gently displace the skin and subcutaneous tissue up or down on the trunk and evaluate the responses. It is helpful to demonstrate the technique on the patient's face. It is not only accuracy but speed that determines the correct response.

The pulp of the finger is more sensitive to touch than pinprick so it is better to test pinprick proximal to the nail.

Proprioceptive sensations

Position sense and sense of passive movement

Position sense of a whole limb or a component requires a sense and awareness of the body map. There is also recognition of internal space. Position sense is a higher sensory compilation of information derived from joints, tendons and muscles that is combined with awareness of the body part as belonging to the patient, which is then compared to the patient's internal map of his or her body parts. This is an elaborated sensation. It can be destroyed at any level of the neuraxis, but is most prominently noted with parietal lobe lesions on the right side.

Parietal copy (Fig. 7.2)

The patient's eyes are closed. The examiner places one hand in a particular position and the patient is asked to copy the posture. Most normal people are extremely good at this maneuver and do it perfectly with one movement. This requires a lot of cortex to perform. The patient must hear and understand the command, which is accomplished by area 22 of the superior temporal gyrus (Wernicke's area). The patient must know right from left (superior parietal lobule), plan the movement (dorsolateral preferential cortex) and, importantly, copy the held position of the hand to a new position. The parietal lobe opposite the moved hand must know this position, and the ipsilateral parietal lobe projects to the motor cortex and signals the position to be copied. Recent information suggests that the right temporal lobe is important for spatial memory. The examiner places fingers of the held hand in different positions and asks the patient to copy them. This tests the integrity of the body map as well as position sense of the fingers. In any patient with an organic brain syndrome this is too complicated a task because of apraxia. A simple way to test pure position sense of the arm is to have the patient close the eyes and then the examiner flexes the ipsilateral arm and observes the patient's ability to copy the position. A similar set of maneuvers is done with the leg. Move the leg off the midline and ask the patient to point to his or her big toe. Normally, this is done with less than a 10° deviation.

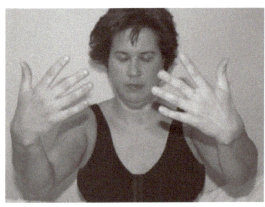

(a)

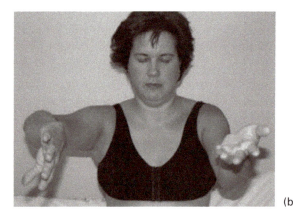

(b)

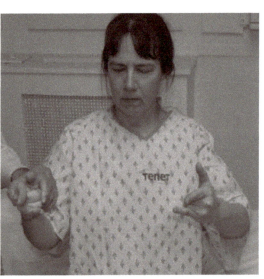

(c)

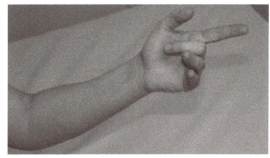

(d)

(e)

Fig. 7.2 Parietal copy. (a) Normal. The examiner places the right hand of the patient in the position shown and the patient copies it quickly and correctly. The hand and arm are moved and hence this is dynamic posture copy. (b) The examiner places the right hand in the position shown but the patient is unable to copy this position. The lesion could be in several places as noted in the text. (c) The examiner extends the index and fifth finger on the patient's right hand with her eyes closed. She is able to copy this posture quickly and accurately with the left hand. The hands are quiet and only the fingers moved. A normal response. (d) The position to be copied (reverse as shown). (e) The patient appears confused and cannot copy the finger posture of the right hand (see text for details).

Sense of passive movement

The distal interphalangeal joint of the index finger or the great toe is moved up and down with the patient's eyes closed. In the hand the patient should be able to detect 1° of flexion or extension and in the great toe 5°. The test is made more difficult by moving the joint slowly. The joint has to be held on the side so that the patient cannot get pressure cues from the skin. If the patient fails the test with the distal intraphalangeal joint it should be repeated at the wrist, ankle, elbow and knee. The sense of passive movement, true proprioception, is keener at more proximal joints. Patients with severe proprioceptive loss from either a lesion of the large neurons of the DRG or the dorsal column have a sense of numbness or heaviness of the extremity that may be difficult to demonstrate objectively. The history reveals that these patients have great difficulty walking or doing anything in the dark.

Vibration sense

This modality is tested with a 128° tuning fork. The fork is struck and then placed in an area of the body that is normal so that the patient can judge the normal sensation. The patient is instructed to close the eyes and then the fork is vibrated and placed on the medial malleolus and lower radius. If there is a gross deficiency, the anterior iliac spine, ribs and clavicle are tested. The test is excellent for localizing a tumor compressing the dorsal columns of the spinal cord. Each vertebral spine is tested from an area of decreased sensibility of the spine to one that is appreciated which may be the level of the mass. Prior to MRI scanning, the procedure was extremely helpful but now these patients would have an MRI scan of the area in question.

In vibration sensibility testing, the patient is asked to report the cessation of the vibration that he or she feels. The examiner may stop the vibration of the tuning fork and notes the time it takes for the patient to recognize the lack of sensation. In general, if it is decreased on the affected side, it will be appreciated for 3–5 seconds more on the unaffected side. If there is a minor abnormality, vibration is not detected when the tuning fork is placed on the abnormal side from the normal side and lasts longer when it is moved from the abnormal to the normal side. Passive movement and vibration sensibility test large fiber sensory loss.

Muscle sensibility

If the root to a muscle is sensitized by any lesion, the deep muscle pain afferents that supply that muscle fire to mechanical pressure. These are deep muscle "C" or A-delta fibers. Normally, only a high threshold or tissue destructive stimulus will discharge them. Thus, if a patient has facet hypertrophy or a disk at S1, and this root is injured, the deep pain afferents that innervate the gastrocnemius muscle fire when the muscle is squeezed and the patient reports pain in the muscle. This form of testing is dramatically helpful in testing for radiculopathy. In this instance, the clinical test is far superior to MRI as this test is very poor in detecting any bony lesion or in demonstrating the relationship of bones to the nerve root. At least 50% of patients with clear radicular motor and sensory defects will have negative MRI scans. Unfortunately, this fact is underappreciated.

Sore muscles can clearly occur from any local process that directly stimulates or sensitizes muscle pain afferents. If muscles are abnormally tender, patients report distress with minimal pressure.

Increased muscle tenderness is common with small fiber polyneuropathies, radiculopathy, myositis and rarely with vitamin B_{12} deficiency. Decreased sensitivity of muscle occurs in syringomyelia, tabes dorsalis and autoimmune destruction of the dorsal root at the entry zone to the spinal cord.

Stereognosis, discriminative sense and graphesthesia

These are abilities dependent both on perception of the object (intact primary modalities) and then on the ability of the brain to build primary sensation into a perception. Hence, these abilities are known as cortical sensation. There is a dramatic interplay in the sensory cortex between movements that stimulate proprioception of the joints, the sensations of touch, pressure and temperature in building a sensory perception. Lesions at all levels of the sensory neuraxis, but primarily the cortex and thalamus, or radiations to the cortex from the internal capsule and corona radiata can cause this type of sensory deficit.

Stereognosis

The patient is asked to close the eyes and a small familiar object is placed into the palm of the patient's hand. A normal person immediately drops the object to the fingertips and then palpates and explores it. The examiner immediately notes deficits in this sphere if the patient has difficulty getting an object out of the palm of the hand. Remember, the patient must have enough primary modality sensation preserved to be able to feel the object. If the patient has difficulty with the hand suspected of the deficit, the object is placed into the normal hand and it is immediately recognized. There are major connections between the parietal lobe and hand areas of the motor cortex, so even the smallest deficit will be noted in the manipulation of the object which is as important as correct identification of the object. Coins are especially useful in this regard. Loss of stereognosis is most helpful in detecting a cortical lesion if other forms of primary sensation are intact or only minimally affected. Thalamic lesions affect all modalities of sensation severely and are capable of destroying vibration sensibility. Parietal lobe lesions are the usual cause of loss of stereognosis. The hand must be able to palpate the object to build secondary sensation.

Two-point discrimination

The two-point discrimination test is the ability of a patient to tell that he or she is stimulated by two blunt stimuli applied simultaneously to adjacent skin areas. The patient is shown how the test is to be carried out by giving him or her the sensory stimulus widely separated. The examiner determines the threshold of the patient to two-point abilities by starting with 1 cm separation of the stimuli and slowly decreasing it to 4–5 mm, which is the threshold on the tip of the index finger. If applied to the lip or tongue patients may have a threshold of 1 mm. On the dorsum of the foot it is 4–5 cm. Patients must have the sensation of light touch intact. An easy way to perform the same maneuver on the body is to touch a spot and ask the patient to touch the same spot. The distance of the error is the two-point discrimination in that area. Patients tend to proximalize the deficits with parietal lobe lesions. Some would argue that touching a spot on the body is a test of body awareness. Another way to test the same phenomenon is to place a diagram of a body in front of the patient and ask him or her to close the eyes. The patient is then touched and asked to place the area of the touch on the diagram with the eyes open. Left parietal deficits cause point localization deficits bilaterally. Right parietal lobe lesions demonstrate deficits on the left side of the body. Two-point discrimination is excellent for determining small deficits. It has been utilized on the fingers, particularly the little finger, for C8 lesions.

Graphesthesia

This is the ability to identify numbers or letters written on the skin surface. The examiner lightly traces the numbers with the forefinger. The easiest number to recognize is three. Frequently, five is the most difficult and seven is often missed or appears difficult to patients. Others feel that 8, 4 and 5 are the easiest. Again, this is objective and is under control of the examiner. It is useful above and below a possible spinal cord sensory lesion. It is most often used to identify a parietal lesion.

Localization of touch and miscellaneous observations

This is a higher cortical sensation and has subtleties. Associated with such is that left parietal lesions may produce bilateral deficits. Surprisingly, there appear to be overlapping sensory maps in the parietal lobe. A patient may have a lesion that interferes with two-point discrimination but not graphesthesia. Rarely, an SI lesion (primary sensory cortex) diminishes all primary modalities of sensation and appears to be a thalamic lesion (Vernet's syndrome). Rarely, an SII lesion (located in the parietal lobe at the foot of SI) abolishes the understanding or perception of pain.

8: Common Patterns of Abnormal Sensation

Total unilateral loss of all forms of sensation

This occurs in the great majority of cases with lesions of the thalamus (ventral posteromedial and posterolateral thalamic nuclei (VPM and VPL)) or as a posterior one-third of the internal capsule lacunar stroke. If this is the case, there is an updrift of the arm with a thalamic hand (adduction and the flexion of the fingers) or a parietal updrift with undulating movement of the fingers (polyminimyoclonus). No extremity moves with normal facility with absent proprioceptive feedback to the motor cortex. There is a loathness to move with thalamic or parietal lesions although strength may be intact. In thalamic lesions, motor function may return prior to complete sensory restitution. Rarely, an SI lesion may cause devastating loss of all primary modality sensation on the contralateral side of the body (Fig. 8.1).

Another site for this sensory deficit is a partial lesion of the thalamus (VPL and VPM primarily), or a lesion of the upper brainstem that occurs in the dorsal pons, but will be accompanied with cranial nerve deficits and a contralateral hemiparesis. If it occurs with a thalamic lesion, the leg is often affected first and the motor deficit most often clears prior to the sensory deficit. At the red nucleus level of the midbrain, a rubral tremor or postural kinetic tremor will be associated. The spinothalamic-mediated sensations of pain and temperature are dorsal to the red nucleus while proprioception and lemniscal sensation are lateral. The third nerve nuclear complex is medial to the red nucleus and in the same arterial territory of the thalamic intrapeduncular artery that arises from the tip of the basilar artery and is often involved by a cardiac embolus. Thus, a third nerve lesion associated with spinothalamic sensory loss would suggest a midbrain lesion.

Unilateral loss of all proprioceptive sensation

This may be caused by a lesion in the thalamic proprioceptive receiving area. There is a particular propensity to have instability while standing and hence a lesion here is often called "ataxia of stance." The area that is involved interrupts proprioceptive pathways from the intermediate zone of the cerebellum, whose origin is the middle cerebellar peduncle. Lesions of the dorsal column nuclei may produce dramatic ataxic oscillations of the arms and leg that may resemble hemiballismus. These movements are usually more prominent in the arms. Gait is wide-based and reeling. The patient is unable to walk in the dark. The vascular territory of the paired posterior spinal arteries are most often compromised to produce the syndrome. Rarely, a foramen magnum tumor or trauma may also cause it.

The most common cause of severe generalized proprioceptive loss occurs with autoimmune attack of the large fibers and neurons of the

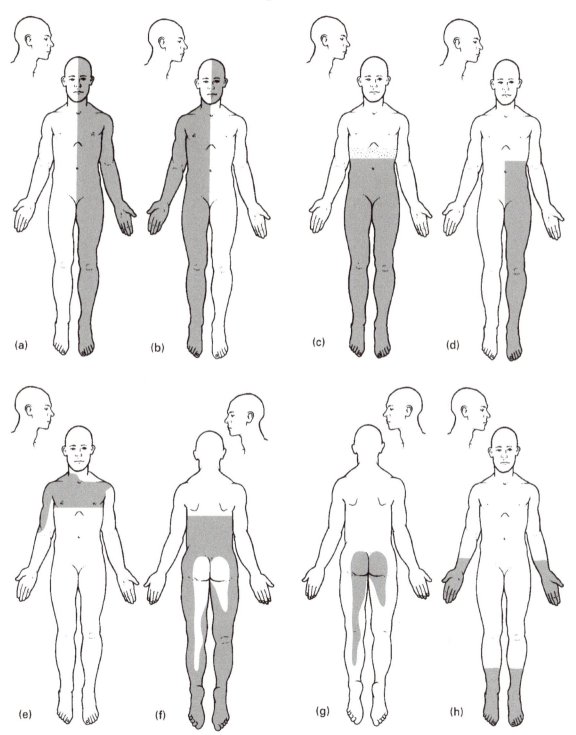

Fig. 8.1 (a) Total hemianalgesia. (b) Lateral medullary. (c) Transverse lesion of the cord. (d) Hemisection. (e) Cuirasse analgesia. (f) Sacral sparing. (g) Saddle anesthesia. (h) Glove and stocking anesthesia. (*Cont'd on page 170*).

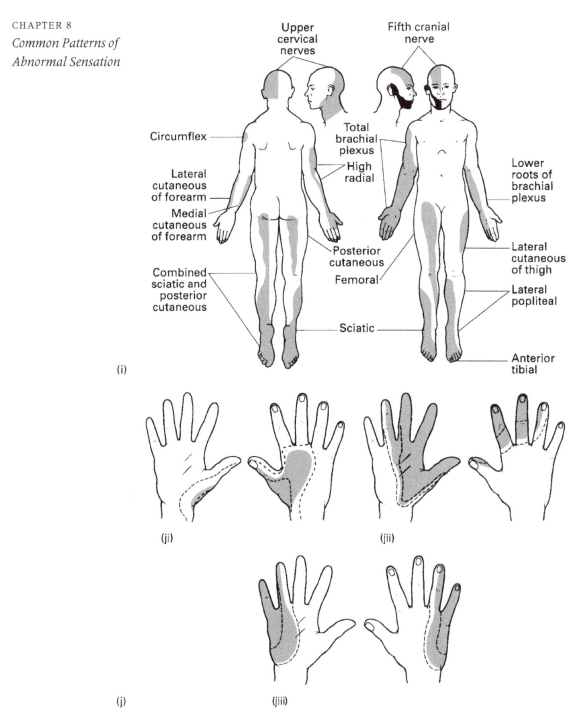

Fig. 8.1 (*cont'd*) (i) Average areas of sensory loss resulting from the more common peripheral nerve lesions. Variation is considerable and in incomplete lesions, the area involved may be greatly reduced. (j) Area supply of: (i) radial; (ii) median; and (iii) ulnar nerves. In each, the shaded area represents the average areas of loss to touch and the lines the degrees of variation dashed that are common. Pain is often lost over less than the smaller area of supply.

dorsal root ganglia (DRG). This is Richter's variant of Guillain–Barré syndrome (GBS). Early tic paralysis may present similarly. Rarely, an upper brainstem infarction affecting lemniscal pathways in the dorsal pons or upper brainstem lateral to the red nucleus causes the syndrome.

Unilateral loss of position sense and cortical sensation, with disturbance of light touch and the quality of pain

These sensory findings are characteristic of a lesion of the thalamic radiations as they ascend to the cortex. The closer the lesion is in the radiation (from the posterior one-third of the posterior limb of the internal capsule) the more dense the primary modality loss of sensation and the more modalities affected. Parietal superficial lesions may affect one modality to a greater degree than others. Central pain occurs following strokes and other lesions of the spinothalamic system anywhere in its course but is often seen when the thalamic parietal radiations are affected. It occurs in 10% of stroke patients.

Unilateral hyperalgesia and hyperesthesia (Fig. 8.2)

Severe augmentation of pain is manifested in several ways. It is common after peripheral root, plexus or nerve injury and is widely missed. In short, root, plexus and nerve injury excite "C" fibers and A-delta fibers. A constant barrage from either direct nerve injury (injury potentials), poorly healed fracture sites or brachial plexus traction injury sets in motion a great number of molecular biologic changes in the DRG cells (particularly the small neurons that encode pain) as well as all pain projecting neurons throughout the neuraxis. The chronic barrage releases glutamate on dorsal horn *N*-methyl-D-aspartate (NMDA) receptors that initiate these molecular biologic changes through calcium mechanisms. These changes cause central sensitization, a state in which peripheral receptive fields enlarge so that pain is not localized to a specific root, plexus or nerve but may be felt on a whole side of the body. This process results in mechanoallodynia, in which an innocuous mechanical stimulus is perceived as painful, as well as hyperalgesia, in which a simple pinprick causes far too much pain for the stimulus applied, and hyperpathia. This condition is the most severe of all pain states. It is harder to appreciate pain, but once this occurs, the pain reaches maximal intensity too quickly, is overwhelming and lasts after the stimulus is withdrawn. This is the basis of chronic regional pain syndrome (CRPS) which is associated with:

1　autonomic dysregulation manifested by increased sweating and poor circulation to the affected part;

2　a movement disorder consisting of difficulty in initiating simple movements, spasms, tremors, increased reflexes and dystonia;

3　swelling;

4　atrophy and dystrophy of the affected part.

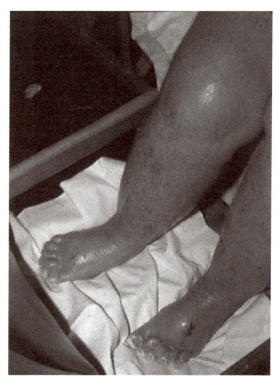

(a)

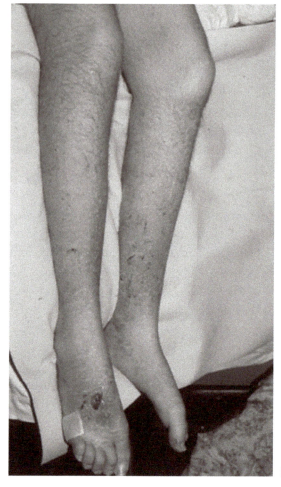

(b)

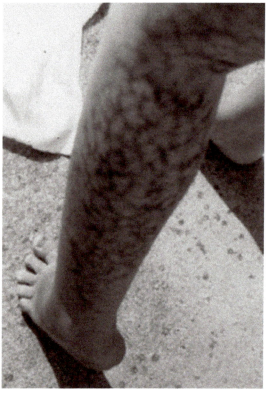

(c)

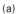

Fig. 8.2 Chronic regional pain syndrome. (a) Severe neurogenic edema noted in patient's right leg. Process is spreading to the left leg. (b) Following diuresis. Severe muscle atrophy is evident. (c) Livedo reticular of the skin. Manifestation of autonomic dysregulation.

This syndrome occurs in 2% of all accidents. The molecular biology of it is becoming clearer and newer treatments are available. It is often missed in its early stages when it is most amenable to treatment. It occurs after central lesions in approximately 10% of patients.

Loss of pain and temperature on one side of the face and opposite side of the body

This is most often the result of occlusion of the vertebral or posterior inferior cerebellar artery whose origin is the vertebral artery. It occurs because the ipsilateral descending sensory tract of the fifth nerve is involved concomitantly with the ascending spinothalamic tract that had crossed at its origin (the spinal segment) from the other side of the body. These patients often complain of a punctate paresthetic feeling in the face ("salt and pepper" paresthesia). The fifth nerve (carrying pain and temperature) crosses and ascends to the ventromedial nucleus of the thalamus in the ventrotegmental spinothalamic tract. A midline medullary lesion may thus cause bilateral facial sensory loss. The spinothalamic tract is laminated with sacral and leg fibers more lateral than trunk, arm and face fibers. Thus, a more lateral lesion of the medulla causes a decrease of pain and temperature in the ipsilateral face and the contralateral sacrum and leg. As the infarction spreads medially, the trunk and arm may be involved. Rarely, during recovery from this type of infarction the sacrum and leg may have recovered and the trunk and arm are involved. If on the left side (chest pain) it has been ascribed to a myocardial infarction. Trunk sensory awareness is more characteristic of spinothalamic tract rather than lemniscal sensory lesions.

Bilateral complete sensory loss below a definite level

This is the hallmark of a spinal cord lesion. Detecting the level of the lesion may be difficult at times. A good way to start is to use a cold tuning fork gently ascending from an area of numbness to an area that the patient can feel. This is followed by a pin in the same manner. Double simultaneous sensory discrimination often demonstrates the lesions in an objective manner as the patient will not report the stimulus in an area of decreased sensibility when he or she is touched above and below the level of altered sensibility. Testing skin proprioception, where the patient is asked to identify if the skin is pushed up towards the nose or down toward the toes, is also very helpful. Using a tuning fork on each dorsal spine is helpful in identifying a spinal cord level if the lesion is dorsal. If the spinal cord lesion is dorsal, vibration sensibility tends to be lost early although it is also carried in the neospinothalamic tract and the tract of the lateral cervical nucleus (upper extremities). If the lesion is at a spinal level, the sensory loss should be two segments lower on the abdomen than the back. In practice, a great number of cervical cord lesions present as a sensory loss at T4–T6 because of the lamination of the spinothalamic tracts (STT). Sacral sparing occurs because of the STT lamination and the dorsal position of sacral fibers in the posterior columns. Rarely, bilateral lower leg sensory loss can occur from a ventral cervical cord lesion. If only pain and temperature are involved the lesion is in the ventral spinal cord. This is usually infarction of the anterior spinal artery, viral myelitis or disk compression. Primary lemniscal sensory loss (posterior column sensation of vibration and position sense) occurs from dorsal spinal cord compressive lesions, Sjögren's syndrome, vitamin B_{12} deficiency and autoimmune processes that affect the large cells of the DRG with secondary posterior column degeneration. In the past, tabes dorsalis was notorious for a "stamping gait" sensory ataxia resulting from large fiber sensory root entry zone defects.

An important differential point between a dropped level resulting from lamination of sensory tracts and a spinal lesion at the segmental level is hyperesthesia close to the level of injury. This is a complicated issue as there are many central changes that occur in pain processing following both peripheral nerve and spinal injuries. The zone of hyperesthesias at the upper level of the spinal injury is often secondary to disinhibition of dorsal horn central pain projecting neurons or irritation of the entering dorsal root nociceptive fibers. This problem is encountered most often with cervical and thoracic cord injuries from motor vehicle accidents, blunt trauma or knives and bullets.

Unilateral loss of pain and temperature sensation below a definite level

This condition is most often seen from a vertical hemisection of the spinal cord. This occurs with knife and bullet injuries to the cord, demyelinating disease and after spinal cord irradiation. In this instance, approximately 1 year after at least 3000 rad have been delivered to the cord a proliferative endarteritis is initiated by the X-ray therapy which obliterates a ventral sulcal artery. Patients present with vibration and proprioceptive loss ipsilaterally under the level of the injury with a contralateral loss of pinprick, pain and temperature. There is paralysis below the level of the lesion on the side of the proprioceptive deficit and 1–2 segments of analgesia at the level of the lesion. This constellation of signs and symptoms is the Brown–Séquard syndrome.

Impairment of pain and temperature sensation over several segments with normal sensation above and below the deficit

This is a central cord lesion that affects the spinothalamic crossing fibers from Rexed Layers I–II of the substantia gelatinosa and those axons from Rexed Layer V at the base of the dorsal horn. If the lesion extends posteriorly, proprioceptive loss occurs in addition because of destruction of the middle layers III–IV of the dorsal horn. This occurs most frequently with syringo-myelia, intrinsic cord tumors, trauma (central cord injury) and cavernous hemangioma of the cord. It must be borne in mind that loss of sensation over many segments (T2–S2) may occur from extrinsic lesions because pressure may compress the blood supply to the cord differentially.

Loss of sensation of "saddle" type

This loss of sensation corresponds to the external skin areas that are involved if the patient was on a saddle (i.e., the lowest sacral dermatomes). If the cauda equina is involved (the lumbar and sacral roots that have left the cord and are coursing downward toward their exit foramina), perineal sensation is involved. This type of lesion is asymmetric, painful, affects all modalities of sensation and is accompanied by sphincter involvement, weakness and loss of reflexes. It is most often caused by a central disk protrusion, trauma, lymphoma and now in a setting of HIV, cytomegalovirus (CMV) infection. If touch is preserved, the lesion is in or near the conus medullaris. The figures contrast sacral sparing with loss of perineal sensation.

Conus medullaris

Conus medullaris lesions (the sacral spinal cord segments at the vertebral level of L1) are characterized by early sphincter and sexual dysfunction, are painless and often cause saddle anesthesia. Epiconal lesions (T11–T12) cause an extensor plantar sign (Babinski's) with preserved knee jerks. Lesions of this area of the cord would be further evaluated by utilizing the bulbocavernous reflex (a pinch of the glans penis causes contraction of the bulbocavernosus muscle behind the scrotum).

Thalamic sensory loss

The thalamus is the locus of the dawn of sensation. Patients who have had a hemispherectomy can feel sensation on the contralateral side of the body. It is hard to localize, there is a delay between the applied stimulus and its perception as well as a loss of all discriminative or elaborated aspects of the modality.

The characteristics of a thalamic sensory loss are its strict adherence to the midline of the body. It is as if a line bisected the patient. The umbilicus seems to have a dual representation as a thalamic lesion may cause bilateral sensory loss around the umbilicus. All modalities are affected including vibration, which is never lost in cerebral SI deficits. A thalamic lesion may split the forehead to vibration even though this is a single bone. This property has to do with neglect or possible inhibition of the sensory cortex. Characteristic of a thalamic lesion may be loss of sensation of all fingertips. The ventroposterior inferior nucleus is usually involved, which receives input from each finger. Thalamic lesions cause bilateral intraoral sensory loss resulting from the bilateral innervation of VPM. Neglect of a sensory stimulus may occur with thalamic lesions, but not to the same extent as with parietal cortex lesions (particularly of the right side). The hand drift of a thalamic patient features adduction of the thumb and flexion of the wrist; that from the parietal lobe is an updrift with finger motion (polyminimyoclonus). A patient with a thalamic lesion often is found in an awkward position in bed (the arm may be askew under the body). Right-sided parietal lesions are often associated with neglect of both near and far space so that the patient is at an angle over to the right side of the bed.

Cortical sensory loss

The parietal lobe is central to somatosensory function, awareness of intrapersonal (that which the individual can touch) and extrapersonal space (that which the individual cannot touch) and awareness of the body parts in space. There is great parietal lobe influence on movements. The left parietal lobe is vital for reading, writing and receptive speech. The right parietal lobe is central to visuospatial processing. Lesions of the primary somatosensory cortex areas 3, 1, 2 (SI) cause specific discriminative sensory defects. A severe lesion of SI causes loss of all modalities of sensation (pain to a minimal degree) and may appear to be a thalamic lesion (Vernet's syndrome). Rarely, a lesion of SII (the foot of SI) causes an inability to appreciate pain.

General parietal lobe higher cortical sensory processing that can be accomplished by both sides of the brain are:
1 two-point discrimination;
2 graphesthesia;
3 localization of body parts in space;
4 stereognosis;
5 point localization on the body surface;
6 the ability to appreciate simultaneous stimuli;
7 simultagnosia (the ability to perceive different components of an object as a whole).

Detailed analysis of parietal lobe function reveals that the posterior parietal cortex areas 7a and 7b are important for reaching and grasping while the anterior superior portion is more important for manipulation and active touch. This area appears to be specialized to utilize stereoscopic vision for fine hand movements. The ventromedial parietal cortex is specialized to recognize gestures or objects (area 7). The inferior parietal lobule is important in the memory or recognition of spatial position. Medial parietal lobe lesions cause a loss of sense of direction.

In any clinical practice the neglect of visual space to the left side of a body part is very strong evidence of a right parietal lesion. It must be remembered that a patient must have adequate somatosensory input to perceive the stimulus presented. All lesions of sensory systems cause some loss of primary modality sensation so that the examiner must decide if the extra dimension of neglect is out of proportion to the expected deficit. There is also an apparent inner gyroscope for the relation of the body to a vertical axis, the subjective visual vertical (SVV). This is manifest by a patient who continues to lean to one side during the examination and actively tries to push his or her body to the midline. Right parietal lobe lesions (behind the primary sensory cortex) cause deficits of the following:

1 Visuospatial processing, which is manifest as the inability to draw a clock or flower correctly (neglecting to fill in the petals or numbers to the left side).

2 Asomatognosia (denial of a body part), the part often assuming a negative quality ("Get that arm out of my bed").

3 Denial of illness (anosognosia), the paralyzed arm and leg claimed to be normal ("I used it yesterday and today I am resting it").

4 Simultagnosia, inability to put together components of an article to perceive it as a whole ("That is an eye, nose and mouth") but no realization that the parts comprise a face. The reverse also can occur. An object may break apart and cannot be maintained as a whole.

5 Left visual neglect.

6 Aprosody, abnormal rhythm of speech.

7 Constructional apraxia, inability to copy the construction of a simple object (matches to construct a flat square design).

8 Dressing apraxia, the patient only putting the right arm in the shirt or trying to put both legs in the right pants leg.

9 The ability to judge the directional orientation of lines, right posterior parietal lesion.

10 The ability to discriminate unfamiliar and familiar faces.

The left parietal lobe is primarily specialized for speech. Patients with posterior lesions demonstrate multiple deficits in this sphere, which is discussed later. The sensory deficit is a bilateral problem with point localization, as well as that of parietal modalities.

Peripheral sensory loss

The nerve roots

In the upper extremities, most mechanical injury of nerve roots occurs at motion segments. These are primarily C5–C6 and C6–C7. If a fusion is performed at C5–C6 (surgical or rarely congenital as in the Klippel–Feil syndrome), C4–C5 becomes a motion segment. C8–T1 never becomes a motion segment and is only involved with severe trauma, obstetric catastrophe or malignancy. In the lower extremity, L5–S1 is the primary motion segment and bears the brunt of life. L4–L5 is also frequently involved in the degenerative arthritic conditions that affect the human spine. As a general rule, besides disk disease, involvement of L1–L3 should suggest medical causes of root involvement such as diabetes mellitus, collagen vascular disease, metastases or lymphoma.

This area of clinical neurology is frequently performed very poorly because clinicians do not know the specific radiations of the common roots, their unusual radiations and the patterns of radiations from brachial and cervical plexus lesions. The following rules make life very easy.

Root involvement of the upper extremity rarely radiates to the hand. C5–C6 disease most often causes pain in the shoulder. C6 may radiate to the lateral forearm. There is no C5 in the hand. C6 rarely radiates to the thumb and index finger. C7 radiates with C6 down the spinous process and slightly medial to it. Very rarely it radiates to the long finger. It does radiate to the triceps. There is no T1 in the hand, it starts at the wrist. C8 innervates the skin of the fourth and fifth finger. Mechanical processes such as disk disease or spondylolisthesis and spondylosis do not radiate to the fourth and fifth finger. This is a very common surgical mistake as many patients are operated upon for C5–C6 disks while the clinical picture points to C8–T1 involvement of the lower trunk of the brachial plexus. If a patient has clear radiation of pain or paraesthesias into the hand, the process is almost always nerve or brachial plexus not radicular.

In the lower extremity, radicular pain frequently radiates to the toes in contrast to the upper extremity. The major levels of involvement are L5–S1. The major movement segments are L5–S1 followed by L4–L5. The L5 root has major differentiating features. In a patient who has severe disease of L5, all components of the root's radiations may be felt. It is much more characteristic of root disease to vary in its radiations. L5 also radiates to the belt line, the buttock, lateral thigh, posterior popliteal fossa, anterior leg, dorsum of the foot to the great toe. It innervates the medial sole of the foot (medial plantar nerve). Other common radiations are to the hip and top of the thigh. The recurrent nerve of Spurling is the dural innervation of L5 and projects to the top of the thigh both as paresthesias and pain. This is a projected radiation into L1–L2 territory. Animal studies in rats have demonstrated that this dural L5 root has anatomic connections to the L1–L2 DRG so there is convergence at this level which is projected to the anterior thigh. Rarely, L5 projects to the scrotum.

The S1 root causes pain in the low back that radiates over the sacroiliac joint to the sciatic notch. In some patients, there is a clear medial gluteal fold radiation. It often radiates into the groin, which is frequently misidentified as a hernia. It is then noted in the lateral posterior thigh (medial posterior thigh is S2) to the posterior popliteal fossa, gastrocnemius muscle, lateral foot and small toe. It innervates the lateral sole of the foot (lateral plantar nerve).

The L4 root innervates the medial leg below the knee to the ankle. Lesions of this root sometimes present as a band around the ankle. L5–S1 is most often involved together as are L4–L5. This is a result of involvement of the root at its exit foramina as well as involvement of the higher root prior to its exit. Only a lateral disk or an osteophyte in the exit foramina involves the root selectively.

Root pain most often is a strip pain. The roots may radiate to the proximal or distal innervation zones, but rarely to both concomitantly. Thus, L5–S1 back disease may be felt solely as pain in the top of the foot or great toe. The hip radiation is commonly involved along with the lateral thigh. S1 frequently radiates to the groin and thigh. Rarely, S1 can be distinctly felt at the tip of the penis or on one side of the vagina. It is difficult to convince an elderly patient that the source of the foot pain is the back. Orthopedists have a difficult time with the L5 radiation into the hip, and it can be hard to convince a general surgeon that the groin pain they witness is from the S1 radiation and not a hernia.

Facet pain comes from involvement of a small branch of the posterior root that exits dorsally immediately after the root clears the exit foramina. It innervates a small 2.5-cm zone lateral to the spinous process.

Pain in the sciatic notch is caused by sensitization of the nerve as it exits into the leg (the nervi nervorum of the nerve sheath) and not the pyriformis muscle syndrome. If the patient is sitting on a hard bench (praying for several hours) we may see the sciatic nerve sensitized in this area, but most often the problem will be found in the back.

The sacroiliac joint gets a great deal of attention and injections. It is a strong joint and nothing much happens to it unless the patient suffers ankylosing spondylitis. The usual pain noted by the patient in this joint again emanates from S1 involvement in the back.

Brachial plexus sensory loss (Figs 8.3 and 8.4)

This sensory loss is rarely diagnosed correctly and is extremely common. The brachial plexus is comprised of the C4–T1 nerve roots. It is anatomically connected to the cervical plexus, which comprise the C1–C4 nerve roots as well as the branchial plexus which emanates from the ventral roots of C1–C4.

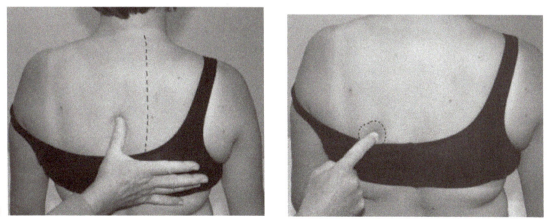

(a)　(b)

Fig. 8.3 Testing the brachial plexus. (a) Shaded area represents the usual back radiations of C6–C7. (b) The tip of the scapula is painful with upper trunk brachial plexus lesions. This pain radiation is known as notalgia. (*Cont'd on page 180*).

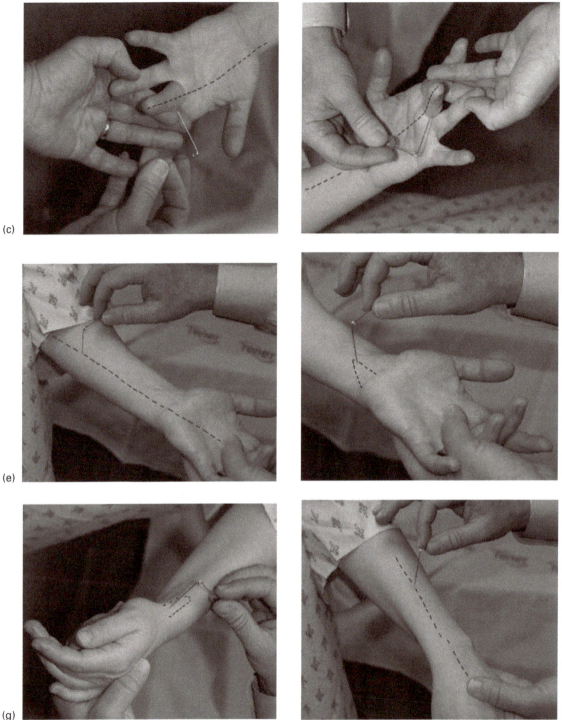

Fig. 8.3 (*cont'd*) (c) The lateral cord splits the third finger on the radial side and encompasses the thumb and index finger. (d) The medial cord splits the third finger to the ulnar side and encompasses the fourth and fifth finger and medial forearm. (e) The lower trunk innervates the entire fourth and fifth finger and continues up the forearm. (f) The ulnar nerve splits the fourth finger to the ulnar side and innervates only a small triangular area beyond the wrist.(g) Pure radial nerve sensory distribution. The "snuff box." (h) The dorsal forearm and hand distribution of the dorsal radial sensory nerve that entered the forearm through the arcade of Frohse.

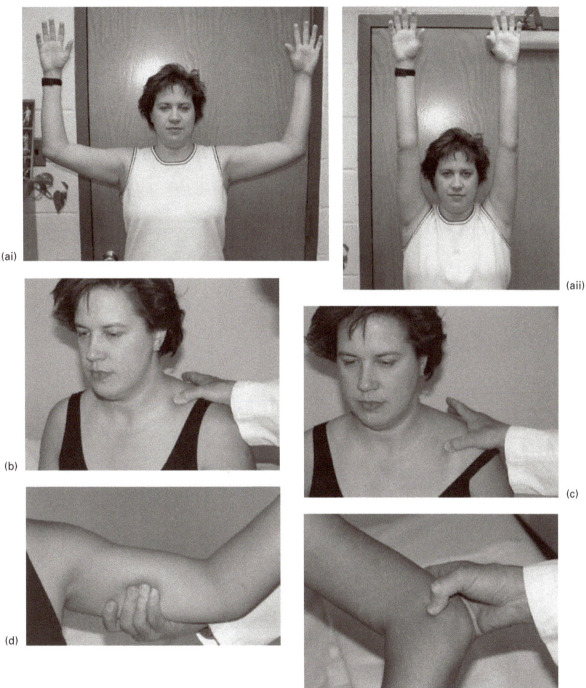

Fig. 8.4 Compression of upper trunk and entire plexus at intraclavicular foss and neurovascular bundle. (ai) Roos' abduction stress maneuver. This maneuver stretches the brachial plexus. A normal person can hold their arms in this position for 3 minutes without parathesias in the fingers. Patients with brachial plexus injuries have parathesias in specific components of the plexus within 30 seconds. (aii) Wright's manuever. This maneuver primarily stretches the upper and lower components of the plexus. (b) The upper trunk of the plexus can be compressed in the supraclavicular fossa. (c) Intraclavicular fossa. The plexus passes between the clavicle and first rib at this point. (d) The neurovascular bundle. The plexus can be compressed against the medial humerus here. (e) Arcade of Frohse. The entrance of the dorsal radial sensory and posterior interosseous nerve into the forearm. (*Cont'd on page 182*).

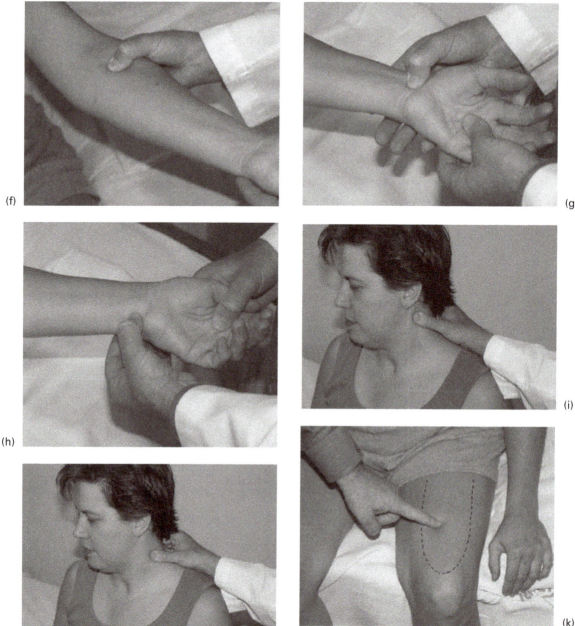

Fig. 8.4 (*cont'd*) (f) The pronator canal. The median nerve enters the forearm between the heads of the muscle and a tight aponeurosis. (g) The carpal tunnel. The median nerve maybe sensitized from higher lesions in the brachial plexus. (h) Guyon's canal. The ulnar nerve lies next to the periform bone at this point. (i) C2. The examiner compresses the exit foramina at C2. The patient often complains of pain at the point of compression which radiates into the neck and face. (j) Spurling's maneuver at C3–C4. If these roots are sensitized, patients complain of pain at the point of compression which radiates to the ear and posterior cervical area (posterior auricular nerve distribution). (k) This is dural radiation of L5. It is frequently mistaken for L1–L3 nerve roots. Frequently, positive along with hip pain, posterior popliteal pain and parasthesias of the great toe.

Clinicians forget that nerves and plexuses slide with extremity and trunk movement. If a nerve root or the plexus is sensitized from prior injury, simple mechanical pressure induced by movement of the extremity will fire nociceptive fibers and cause pain. This is the basis of the straight leg raising (SLR) test in which the sciatic nerve is stretched. Lasègue's maneuver, in which the ankle is dorsiflexed during the SLR test stretches the sciatic nerve further. Lying in bed and having the neck flexed pulls up the lumbosacral roots. If any are sensitized, the involved root becomes painful (Mayo clinic sign). The brachial plexus slides a great deal, at least 1 cm with various movements. No patient with a brachial plexus lesion (one that affects its sensory components) will be comfortable with the arms above the head. The Roos' abduction stress maneuver causes pain in that component of the plexus that is involved. Wright's maneuver usually stretches both the upper and lower trunks of the plexus. The divisions of the plexus are not clinically helpful.

The pain from an upper trunk lesion (composed of the C5–C6 roots) radiates across the trapezius ridge and down the medial scapular border. C6–C7 radiculopathy radiates directly down the spine. The lateral cord sensory distribution is the lateral foramen and includes the thumb, index and radial side of the third finger. Medial cord sensory distribution is the medial forearm and the ulnar side of the third, fourth and fifth finger. The intercosticobrachial nerve takes origin from the medial cord and innervates the skin of the lateral chest wall, under the breast to the xiphoid. The superior branch of the nerve innervates the anterior chest wall. Radiations of pain from this nerve, particularly if noted on the left side, are misdiagnosed as coronary disease or pulmonary disease. The xiphoid component of the nerve radiation is misdiagnosed as acid reflux or ulcer disease. If on the right, costothoracic margin radiations are misdiagnosed as gallbladder disease. The superior division is often misdiagnosed as costochondritis. Of course, anything around the breast in a woman is misdiagnosed as breast cancer. This nerve causes more misdiagnosis than any other in the human body.

The middle trunk posterior cord plexus radiations are on the dorsal portion of the upper arm. They radiate along the triceps muscle. The dorsal sensory radial nerve, the sensory extension of the middle trunk posterior cord enters the forearm through the arcade of Frohse (medial to the lateral epicondyle) to innervate the dorsal forearm and extensor surface of the thumb, index and third finger).

The upper trunk of the plexus is most easily palpated in the supraclavicular fossa. The supraclavicular notch and at the tip of the scapula is also usually painful. The radiation to the tip of the scapula is notalgia. It must be remembered that gallbladder pain radiates to the same distribution. The cords of the plexus can be compressed laterally at the costoclavicular junction and against the medial humerus. The median nerve enters the forearm at the pronator canal in the antecubital fossa, the sensory component of the radial nerve through the arcade of Frohse and the ulnar nerve through the cubital tunnel. If they are sensitized because of lesions of the plexus from which they originate, compression will produce a prominent Tinel's sign as they enter the forearm. The pain will only be felt at the area of compression. Severe sensitization will cause radiation of pain in the entire cord distribution.

Radiations of the cervical plexus

The sensory components of the cervical plexus arise from the dorsal roots of C2–C4. There is no skin representation of C1. The dorsal roots of C2–C3 form the preauricular nerve which overlaps V2 and V3. Patients complain of a dull ache in this distribution and abnormal sensitivity and pain is frequently associated with neurogenic edema. There is hyperemia and swelling in the nerve distribution from release of vasoactive neuropeptides on the blood vessels of the face. The two most active neuropeptides are substance P (SP), which produces capillary leakage, and calcitonin gene-related peptide (CGRP), which paralyzes the smooth muscles of the blood vessels. The pain is a chronic aching, as opposed to the lancinating pain of tic douloureux, which only lasts for 10–15 seconds at most. The posterior roots of C3 and C4 form the posterior auricular nerve that innervates the posterior occiput, the mastoid, most of the pinna and the posterior parietal area. The lesser occipital nerve innervates the lower posterior occiput while the greater occipital innervates the more anterior parietal areas of the calvarium. C2 frequently projects to the brow. The seventh nerve innervates the mastoid bone and some of the external auditory canal. V2 innervates the pre tragus. It is common for a C2 radiation to be most prominent over the brow (typical for a spondylitic headache). Most pain in the back of the head and face is from the cervical plexus rather than cervical nerve roots. The pain of temporomandibular joint (TMJ) only radiates to the mid parietal areas, jaw and neck. It is not unusual to see root cervical plexus and TMJ pain combined in younger patients. If the cervical and branchial plexus are involved, patients frequently complain of difficulty swallowing. The exact complaint is that food is "stuck in my throat." This is secondary to spasm of the cricopharyngeus muscle (the external esophageal sphincter) and dyssynergia of the posterior pharyngeal muscles (tenth cranial nerve) that pushes the bolus to the cricopharyngeus muscle that fails to open rapidly enough. This is a component of the movement disorder of CRPS.

Glove and stocking anesthesia

As a general rule, a metabolic dying back neuropathy causes loss of sensation in the feet that gradually ascends. Once the numbness is perceived above the knee, patients start to notice sensory changes in the fingers and hands. In severe neuropathies, the middle part of the chest is numb (a shield distribution), the nerves are dying back from the spinal dorsal root ganglia. The mid face is numb from dying back of the fifth nerve. This form of distal to proximal sensory loss is characteristic of metabolic and toxic neuropathies. Different fiber sizes mediate different sensory modalities. Small fiber neuropathies such as those caused by paraneoplastic processes (anti-Hu antibody mediated), amyloid (transthyretin met 30) and antisulfatide antibodies characteristically burn. Large fiber (A alpha), 12–22 μm, that mediate vibration and proprioceptive sensation are noted with vitamin B_{12} deficiency, diphtheria and some hereditary motor sensory neuropathies. The large fiber neuropathies have concomitant loss of reflexes while in small fiber neuropathy they are preserved. Rarely, an incomplete cervical cord lesion such as multiple sclerosis or compression can present with a stocking glove distribution.

The loss of all forms of sensation over a clearly defined part of the body is caused by a complete root or peripheral nerve lesion. There are few complete sensory neuropathies, but a posterior root lesion (usually surgical) will be. Mononeuritis multiplex, which is a vasculitis of the blood supply to a nerve, causes multiple successive large nerve injury (median, ulnar, femoral). Diabetes, systemic lupus erythematosus (SLE), periarteritis fossa as well as cancer and trauma are the most common causes.

Loss of vibration sense alone

This is a normal concomitant of aging that is most notable in the lower extremities. It also occurs with intrinsic spinal cord lesions, multiple sclerosis and syringomyelia. In the latter, the syrinx is lateral, which affects the pathways from the lateral cervical nucleus rather than the dorsal columns.

Loss of position and vibration sense alone

This occurs with a lesion of the posterior columns or their nuclei at C1–C2. The primary clinical manifestation is proprioceptive loss. If the process happens acutely from infarction of the posterior medullary arteries or compression at the foramen magnum, patients may have wild flailing movements of the arms and a severe lateral drift of the outstretched arms. The process occurs with tabes dorsalis, Friedreich's ataxia, carcinomatous neuropathy, the Richter's variant of GBS, vitamin B_{12} deficiency, the cervical myelopathy associated with HIV and Sjögren's syndrome. If there is a clear level of involvement there is usually compression of the posterior spinal cord. Cervical stenosis, Chiari malformation or foramen magnum stenosis that occurs with achondroplasia are other causes of central loss of position and vibration sensibility. The peripheral involvement of the DRG in autoimmune disease or from chemotherapy are increasingly being recognized.

Loss of specific nerve sensation of the extremities

Patchy sensory loss

Irregular or patchy sensory loss occurs with intrinsic spinal cord lesions (often secondary venous infarction from compression and blockage of venous outflow) such as tumor or vascular malformation. This occurs with recovery from a Brown–Séquard lesion and that from spinothalamic involvement in Wallenberg's syndrome. Leprosy and other polyneuropathies that involve unmyelinated C fibers in the skin may also give the same picture. Loss of sensation in the face (onion skin pattern), forearm, lower legs and hands as well as ovoid areas on the trunk (Hitzig's spots) were seen in the past with tabes dorsalis.

Intercostal (one or two segment loss) suggests diabetes, herpes zoster and rarely carcinoma of the lung. Hyperalgesia (a painful stimulus is perceived as too painful) occurs with posterior root, root entry zone or with CRPS types I and II. A recovering nerve demonstrates uneven return of modality and distribution of sensation.

Sensory loss in the face

Most clinicians ascribe sensory loss in the face to tic douloureux or sinus disease. The major abnormalities that affect the face do so in particular patterns. Both the patient and the physician are delighted with the diagnosis of sinus disease as a cause of facial pain. This is most often incorrect unless the patient has obvious pain over the frontal and maxillary sinuses or postnasal drip and a cough. Varieties of migraine in the young, a brow headache from cervical spondylosis in the elderly and preauricular nerve radiations from the cervical plexus make up the great core of facial pain rather than tic douloureux or sinus disease.

Migraine is inextricably associated with the fifth cranial nerve both in pathogenesis and in the distribution of sensory abnormality. It is clearly associated with mechanoallodynia (an innocuous touch stimulus is perceived as painful) in a distribution of the fifth nerve. Many migraine patients suffer mechanoallodynia of the V2–V3 distribution. Most often, migraine is associated with pain in the V1 distribution. This has been well described by Raeder and may be associated with a Horner's syndrome. Cluster migraine has all of the features of migraine, but the pain is in or behind the eye to a great extent. SUNCT is a recently described syndrome that is defined by sudden unilateral neuralgiform pain associated with conjunctival injection and tearing. Most migraine patients complain of pain with extraocular movement (behind the eyes) associated with photophobia and phonophobia. Paroxysmal hemifacial pain is sharp, occurs many times during the day for a few seconds with each occurrence often in a V2–V3 distribution. It is exquisitely sensitive to prostaglandin antagonists. Periorbital pain is also encountered frequently with migraine. Pain in the upper inner corner of the eye with a severe boring quality may trigger migraine and is caused by trochlear muscle irritation.

A headache between the eyes suggests pituitary disease, anterior communicating artery aneurysm and sphenoid sinusitis. The latter may have a radiation to the top of the head. A headache above the eye, but below the brow may be from stretch of the diaphragma sella secondary to a pituitary adenoma. Lateral eyebrow headaches occur from posterior cerebral or vertebral artery disease.

A common radiation of C2, particularly in spondylitic patients, is to the brow. There will be a spondylitic neck posture. Lateral to the eye, headache is from the anterior temporal area, temporal arteritis, middle fossa lesions and occasionally an occipital lobe hemorrhage. The infraorbital nerves innervate the skin under the eye and are frequently damaged from facial fractures or plastic surgery. The supraorbital nerve, which innervates a major part of the brow and the lower part of the forehead, may be injured during cosmetic procedures.

Sinus headaches causes tenderness over the frontal and maxillary sinus, are worse in the morning and then improve with drainage until about 4 PM when they start to recur. They are accompanied by a postnasal drip.

Tic douloureux

This is one of the most striking pains in medicine. It lasts for only 10–15 seconds, may recur many times during the day and most frequently affects the V2 or V3 division of the fifth nerve. The "tic convulsive" is the sharp head movement brought about by the lancinating pain. The trigger zones are in the area of a cat's whiskers. A slight mechanical stimulus of the face, swallowing and chewing are common triggers. There is a refractory period following each jab of pain where the usual trigger stimulus fails to elicit an attack. There is no motor or sensory loss in the fifth nerve division that is affected. If there is a postural component, the patient may be able to modify the attack by placing his or her head in a particular position. This maneuver suggests that a branch of the anterior inferior cerebellar artery may be touching the nerve.

The headache of temporomandibular joint disease causes pain in the joint itself, radiates to the parietal region and the C3 root distribution of the neck and is associated with jaw deviation and inability to open the mouth fully. It is occasionally associated with tinnitus as the joint is next to the eighth nerve complex (cochlea).

Sjögren's disease and scleroderma often affect the fifth cranial nerve. There is usually numbness in all divisions of the nerve as the primary pathology is the gasserian ganglion. Trichloroethylene and stilbamidine occasionally preferentially affect the fifth nerve nucleus, with consequent numbness of the face.

Chronic regional pain syndrome types I and II

This is a severely painful condition that follows approximately 1–5% of accidents. Almost all nerve injuries can cause the illness, but the median and sciatic are most prominent.

187

The condition has five major components:

1 pain: the special features of which are mechano- and thermal allodynia, hyperalgesia and hyperpathia;

2 neurogenic edema;

3 autonomic dysregulation evidenced by abnormal circulation of the affected area, livedo reticularis and hyperhidrosis;

4 a movement disorder that consists of inability to initiate or maintain movements, dystonia, weakness, spasms and tremors;

5 atrophy and dystrophy.

CRPS type I refers to the syndrome as noted above without an identifiable nerve injury (the C and A-delta fibers are injured in the tissue that is affected) while in CRPS type II an identifiable nerve injury is recognized. The pain is regional and does not respect a root or nerve distribution. It is more severe than expected and may spread to all parts of the body. In its earlier stages, it is often sympathetically maintained, but with time becomes sympathetically independent. Early in the course of the illness the extremity is suffused and hot, but later becomes mottled, cyanotic and cold.

9: The Motor Sensory Links

The reflexes

A successful examination of reflexes requires both the patient and the examiner to be comfortable. The muscle is placed in a comfortable position under slight stretch. The examiner places his or her finger on the major tendon of the muscle and lets the hammer freely fall. The hammer should do most of the work.

The examiner notes three major components of a reflex:

1   its threshold or how easy it is to elicit;

2   the speed in which the antagonist muscle is brought into play (too quickly with spasticity and too late with cerebellar disease);

3   pathologic spread; reflexes should stay at the segmental level.

The gamma loop governs the length of intrafusal fibers of the nuclear bag. These are motor cells in the spinal cord that receive both excitatory and inhibitory influences and determine tone. The nuclear bag is in parallel with the long axis of somatic muscles and the ease with which the intrafusal fibers fire the annulospiral endings that depolarize the anterior horn cell determines the threshold of the reflex. Thus, actively firing gamma neurons in the spinal cord cause the intrafusal fibers to shorten, increase the afferent barrage from annulospiral endings and partially depolarize anterior horn cells. Thus, when the volley of afferent synapses is excitatory to these anterior horn cells they fire very easily (a low threshold). If there is poor inhibition in the spinal cord because of degeneration of the corticospinal tracts above the segment that is tested, or lack of supranuclear inhibition of these gamma neurons, the reflex will not only fire too easily, but will spread to other segments. The engagement of antagonist muscles stops the reflex. This is done by afferent information generated by "flower spray" endings in association with cerebellar and other modulatory influences. A normal reflex, an example being the knee jerk, should elicit 2.5 swings of the leg before it stops. If the threshold to fire the reflex is too low (i.e., it can be elicited by a slight tap of the finger or a flick of the finger) and the antagonist muscles are engaged too easily, the patient has a spastic reflex. The agonist muscle cannot fully complete its action prior to the antagonist muscle being called into play. The tone will be increased and often Babinski's and Hoffman's signs will be elicited. The most common cause of these findings are lesions of the corticospinal pathways. If the antagonists are not called into play, the muscle's primary action will not be modulated correctly, the agonist will extend or flex the extremity through too great an arc and the reflex will be pendular. If we again use the knee jerk as an example, the leg will oscillate back and forth 4.5–5 times before it stops. Associated findings will be a higher threshold to fire the reflex and decreased tone of the affected muscle.

Gamma motor neurons that set tone and alpha motor neurons that fire the agonists and antagonists of specific muscles have to work in concert. In a spastic patient, tone is increased and agonist muscles have to work through the excess tone to effect their function. Normally, gamma neurons are delicately integrated with the agonists they subserve and stop firing with movement, thus lessening tone when that muscle is recruited so it functions easily.

Reflex testing gives the examiner the opportunity to evaluate the patient on a segmental level such as a radicular problem and the general state of the nervous system. Diffuse degenerative processes frequently destroy the motor cortex, thus increasing reflex excitability from lack of inhibition. Excitement may increase reflex excitability by influencing the gamma loop through the reticular formation. Peripheral neuropathies dampen or destroy reflexes because the sensory afferents cannot relay information to the spinal cord and motor axons cannot innervate the muscle. Neuromuscular disease abnormalities may increase reflex excitability of muscle because of spreading acetylcholine sensitivity of the sarcolemmal membrane. As acetylcholine receptors are blocked at the neuromuscular junction by anti-bodies, as is seen with acquired myasthenia, new receptors spread along the muscle surface that render it mechanosensitive. Normally, only chemo-sensitive acetylcholine receptors face muscle afferent fibers. Vibrating the muscle membrane by striking a reflex fires the muscle directly. The reverse occurs with the periodic paralyses. Muscles cannot be fired because of deficits of the sarcolemmal T system and changes of the sarcolemmal mem-brane. They cannot be depolarized by reflex testing.

As a general rule, peripheral neuropathies decrease reflexes. In muscle disease, the reflexes are proportional to the mass of muscle that remains. There are exceptions. In Duchenne muscular dystrophy, the intrafusal fibers of the nuclear bag are affected and the normal afferent drive to anter-ior horn cells is less than normal so that reflexes are often unobtainable. In polymyositis, the inflammation of the process also affects the nuclear bag intrafusal fibers and reflexes may be increased because of partial depo-larization of anterior horn cells fired from irritated annulospiral endings. In radiculopathy, both the sensory and motor arc of the reflex may be blocked at the foraminal exit canal with loss of the affected reflex.

In general, lesions of motor pathways above the spinal level decrease inhibition of anterior horn cells and increase reflexes. This is often helpful in determining the level of a motor lesion. The cortex is biased toward inhi-bition. In a mammalian system, action is required quickly. A spring only has to be released and the organism does not have to ramp up the muscle. A snake has to heat up before it can move. As a general rule, a strictly cortical lesion may increase reflexes because more inhibitory neurons are damaged

Fig. 9.1 Jaw jerk. The patient opens the jaw slightly. The examiner taps down lightly on the forefinger below the lower lip. There is a slight upward jerk of the jaw. If a lesion is above the mid pons, the jaw jerk is hyperactive as are extremity reflexes. Symmetrically exaggerated reflexes of the extremities as well as an increased jaw jerk occurs with pseudobulbar palsy, multiple sclerosis and motor neuron disease. If the jaw jerk is normal but the clavicular biceps reflex is increased, the lesion is between the mid pons and C4.

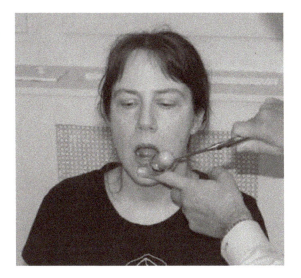

than excitatory ones. The usual teaching is that an acute cortical lesion decreases reflexes for approximately 6 weeks when they then become hyperactive. The deeper a lesion is in the brain the more likely there is to be "brain shock" with depressed reflexes. There are some notable exceptions. Lateral putaminal basal ganglion lesions cause increased reflexes as do lesions of the midbrain (particularly at collicular areas). Early and chronic compressive lesions of the spinal cord are associated with increased reflexes as a result of disinhibition.

The jaw jerk is particularly useful in determining both the segmental level of a problem and the general state of the patient's neuraxis (Fig. 9.1). It depends on proprioceptive and touch information from the masseter muscles that synapse on neurons and interneurons of the fifth nerve nucleus of the mid pons by means of the mesencephalic tract of the fifth nerve. If the jaw jerk is too active, there is loss of inhibition above the mid pons.

It must be remembered that electrolyte imbalance changes the ability of the muscle membrane itself to be depolarized. A high or low sodium and potassium level decrease reflex activity. A low calcium and magnesium level increase muscle membrane activity by increasing membrane excitability.

Pain and emotional stress increase reflex activity through a variety of mechanisms, most of which work through the reticular formation. Some patients are normally hyporeflexive. Reinforcement procedures such as the Jendrassik maneuver, pulling the fingers apart, may then elicit reflexes. Often, clinicians get a reflex and run home without really questioning what it evaluates. It gives the examiner great objective insight into the motor sensory integration of the patient and whether the problem is segmental, structural or metabolic.

The upper limbs (Fig. 9.2)

The easiest way to examine the upper extremity reflexes is to have the patient sit comfortably on the examination table with the arm resting on the lap.

The biceps jerk (see Fig. 9.2a)

The forefinger rests on the biceps tendon in the antecubital fossa. The examiner then hits the forefinger and both feels the tendon contract and the

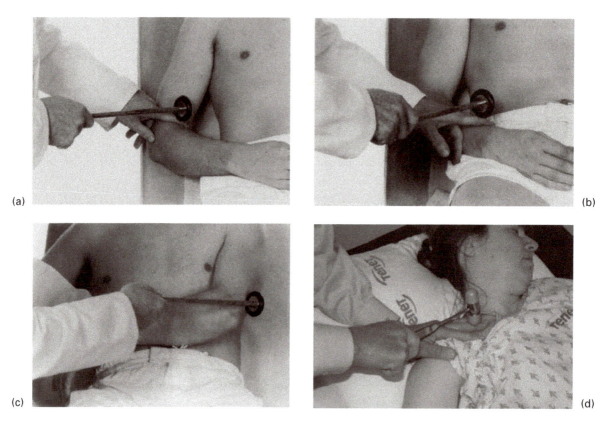

(a)

(b)

(c)

(d)

Fig. 9.2 (a) The biceps jerk. Technique: press the forefinger gently on the biceps tendon in the antecubital fossa and then strike the finger with the hammer. Normal result: flexion of the elbow and visible contraction of the biceps muscle. Segmental innervations: C5. Peripheral nerve: musculocutaneous. (b) The supinator jerk. Technique: strike the lower end of the radium approximately 5 cm above the wrist. Watch the movement of the forearm and fingers. Normal result: contraction of the brachioradialis and flexion of the elbow. The biceps often contracts as well and slight flexion of the finger may occur. Segmental innervations: C5–C6. Peripheral nerve: radial. (c) The triceps jerk. Technique: by holding the patient's hand, draw the arm across the trunk and allow it to lie loosely in the new position. Then strike the triceps tendon 5 cm above the tendon. Normal result: extension of the elbow and variable contractions of the triceps. Segmental innervations: C6–C7. Peripheral nerve: radial. (d) Clavicular biceps. Technique: the examiner places the forefinger on the clavicle and gently taps it and observes the contraction of the biceps. A method to evaluate the excitability of C5–C6. If the jaw jerk is normoactive (mid pons), the lesion should be between the mid pons and C5–C6.

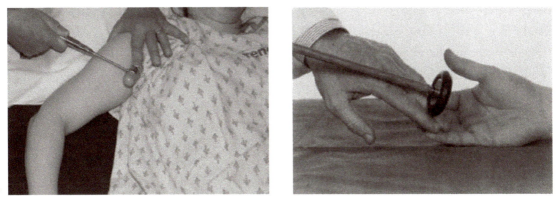

(e)   (f)

Fig. 9.2 (*cont'd*) (e) Pectoral reflexes. Technique: place the tip of the index finger on the pectoral muscle tendon as it forms the anterior margin of the axilla and strike the fingers. Normal result: adduction of the arm and visible contraction of the pectoralis margin. Segmental innervations: C5–T1. Peripheral nerve: lateral and medial pectoral nerves. (f) Finger flexion reflexes. Technique: allow the patient's hand to rest palm upwards, the fingers slightly flexed. The examiner gently interlocks his or her fingers with the patient's and strikes them with the hammer. Normal result: slight flexion of all fingers and of the interphalangeal joint of the thumb. Segmental innervations: C6–T1. Peripheral nerve: median.

forearm flex. The segmental primary innervation is C5 with an overlap of C6. The peripheral nerve innervating the muscles is the musculocutaneous nerve.

The inverted radial reflex is extremely helpful in identifying a cervical lesion at C5–C6. The examiner notes no contraction of the biceps with usual reflex testing, but abnormal finger flexion. Extremely rarely, the patient will have no contraction of the biceps, but contraction of the triceps with extension of the forearm. This occurs because there are two lesions involving the cervical spinal cord. The first is usually at C4–C5, which is compressive (disk, spondylosis or stenosis), which increases excitability at segments below this level and decreases the threshold of the biceps reflex. The second lesion is at the exit foramina of C5–C6 in the cervical cord. When the reflex is attempted the arm is vibrated. Sensory afferent information can enter the cord at C7, C8, T1 as well as C2–C4. It cannot enter the cord at C5–C6 because there is compression of the entire nerve root (motor and sensory) at the C5–C6 exit foramina. Thus, the biceps will not contract because its dorsal root cannot relay sensory information and the ventral root cannot depolarize the muscle. However, all segments of the cord below C4–C5 are disinhibited as a result of a compressive lesion at this level, and the vibration entering the cord at C7, C8, T1 is sufficient to depolarize anterior horn cells at this lower level, which causes extension of the arm (triceps – C7) rather than the expected flexion from biceps contraction at C5. Finger flexion (C8) occurs because these muscles are innervated by anterior horn cells below C4–C5 and the vibration that entered the spinal cord at that level (C8–T1) was sufficient to fire these neurons.

This is not an esoteric phenomenon. All patients over 40 years of age develop cervical and lumbar spondylosis due to the act of living. This occurs at all motion segments of the vertebral column but primarily at C5–C6 and L5–S1. Most examiners view reflex abnormalities as a purely central problem except in disk disease. The condition of the neck determines a great deal of reflex abnormality in an elderly person and must be calculated into the reflex equation. The examiner should always check the mobility of the neck to all planes as well as evaluate it for spondylitic forward flexed posture and other aspects of craniovertebral junction defects usually suggested by an abnormality short neck. Compression from these pathologies increase reflexes because of corticospinal inhibition below the affected segment.

The brachioradialis jerk (see Fig. 9.2b)

The primary roots are C5–C6 and its nerve is the radial. The examiner taps the forefinger, which rests on the radius approximately 5 cm above the wrist. The normal reaction is contraction of the brachioradialis and flexion of the forearm. The reflex can be further magnified by having the patient flex the arms in front and gently tapping the radius while observing the arc of flexion of the forearm.

The triceps reflex (see Fig. 9.2c)

If the patient is sitting, he or she should gently rest the open hand on the quadriceps which places the tendon comfortably in front of the examiner. Both the patient and the examiner are relaxed in this position. Alternatively, the arm can be drawn across the trunk. The segmental innervation is C6–C7 and its peripheral nerve is the radial. The triceps reflex may be the only surviving reflex in Guillain–Barré syndrome (GBS).

The clavicular biceps reflex (see Fig. 9.2d)

The examiner strikes the finger that rests on the clavicle. If the biceps contracts, there is disinhibition above C5–C6. There may be concomitant contraction of the pectoral muscle. If the jaw jerk is normal, the lesion must then be between the mid pons and C4.

The pectoral reflexes (see Fig. 9.2e)

The index finger is placed on the pectoral muscle tendon in the axilla and tapped. There is adduction of the arm and contraction of the pectoralis major muscle. The segmental innervation is the entire plexus from C4–T1. The peripheral nerves are the medial and lateral pectoral nerves.

The finger flexion reflex (see Fig. 9.2f)

The patient's fingers gently rest on the examiner's. The examiner taps the patient's fingers and feels contraction of the fingers against the examiner's own. The interphalangeal joint of the thumb contracts. The segmental innervation is C8–T1. This is a primary component of the lower trunk of the brachial plexus which is hard to assess any other way. The median nerve is the innervation.

The lower limbs (Fig. 9.3)

The patient should be comfortably seated on the edge of the table. The leg should be allowed to oscillate until it stops after the knee is tapped. The foot

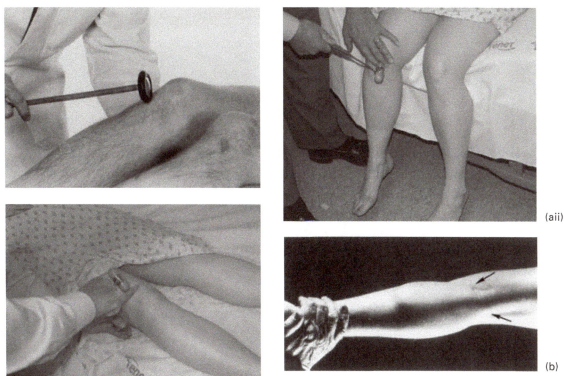

(ai)

(aii)

(aiii)

(b)

Fig. 9.3 (ai) The knee jerk in a bed-bound patient. Technique: the eye should not be too high above the patient's knees, and so if the bed is too low the examiner may have to kneel. To compare the two sides, the left arm (for a right-handed examiner) is placed under both knees in order to flex them together. If the patient holds the legs rigidly, instruct him or her to lie back and let the heels fall on the bed. This often produces complete relaxation. The patella tendon can then be struck lightly on each side, increasing the strength if there is response. A light tap is best for comparing the two sides. Watch the movements of the lower leg and of the quadriceps muscle. Normal result: extension of the knee and visible contraction of the quadriceps. Segmental innervation: L3–L4. Peripheral nerve: femoral. (aii) A method to evaluate the relationship of agonist and antagonist coupling. Increased agonist muscle activity with too rapid check is seen with spasticity. A pendular reflex suggests cerebellar disease. (aiii) A method if the patient cannot bend the knees. Place the finger just above the patella and, while the legs are extended, strike it in a peripheral direction. The quadriceps contract and the patella will be pulled upwards. This method detects slight differences between the two sides and can be used when the lower leg has been amputated. (b) Hamstring reflex. Technique: the patient, lying on the stomach, attempts to flex the knee against resistance. The biceps is seen laterally, the semitendinosus medially. (*Cont'd on page 196*).

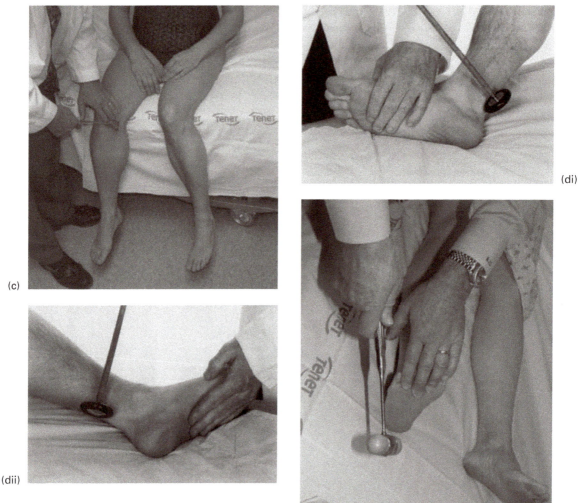

(c)

(di)

(dii)

(diii)

Fig. 9.3 *(cont'd)* (c) Crossed adductor reflex. The examiner taps the right medial tibia. If there is adduction of the left leg disinhibition of the spinal cord above L2 is present or there is generalized disinhibition of the neuraxis. (d) The ankle jerk. (di) Technique. This reflex appears to present technical difficulties, and is frequently recorded as absent when correct technique produces a perfectly normal response. The patient's leg should be externally rotated and slightly flexed at the knee. The examiner uses the left hand to dorsiflex the foot. (dii) For the left leg, the examiner moves to the other side of the bed. The Achilles tendon is then struck and both the movement of the foot and the contraction of the calf muscles are observed. Normal result: plantar flexion of the foot and contraction of the gastrocnemius. Segmental innervation: S1. Peripheral nerve: medial popliteal or sciatic nerve. (diii) Ankle jerk with patient in bed. The examiner dorsiflexes the ankle which stretches the Achilles tendon. This maneuver decreases the threshold to obtain the reflex.

should be evaluated by inspection. If it is dropped, inverted and plantar flexed, there is a segmental lesion of L5–S1. The L4 root is now dominant and the foot is inverted. The same occurs with decortication, upper motor neuron lesions, as well as the primary and secondary dystonias. If the patient is in bed, the examiner instructs him or her to lie flat and rest the legs with the knees flexed on the arms and the patella is struck. The knee should extend and the quadriceps contract. Note is made of the number of oscillations is takes to have the leg cease oscillating as well as how far the arc of the reflex extended the leg and the speed with which the agonist is engaged (the hamstrings). The primary root is L4, but there is a significant contribution from L3. The nerve is the femoral.

An alternate method of eliciting the reflex is to depress the patella with the forefinger and then tap the forefinger. The quadriceps contracts and the patella is pulled upwards.

The hamstring reflex (see Fig. 9.3b)

These are the primary antagonists of the quadriceps and allow for palpation of their tendons. The examiner places the forefinger on the semi-tendinosus tendon which is lateral in the posterior popliteal fossa and taps the tendon. The strength of the contracture is noted and the muscle can be seen to contract. The major root is L5. Similarly, the semimembranosus tendon is tapped and the semimembranosus muscle is seen to contract. This is primarily the L4 root. Both are high sciatic nerve innervations.

The crossed adductor reflex (see Fig. 9.3c)

The examiner places his or her forefinger on the medial side of the tibia at the knee and delivers a sharp tap. The adductor magnus contracts and the thigh is pulled medially. The major root tested is L2 as part of the obturator nerve. The contralateral side should not move. If it adducts and the leg moves medially, there is spinal cord disinhibition above L1–L2.

The ankle jerk (see Fig. 9.3d)

This reflex can be examined by several techniques. The easiest is to have the patient sit on the edge of the bed with the feet dangling. The examiner can then dorsiflex the foot which varies the tension on the Achilles tendon (increases the proprioceptive and tendon afferent input to the L5–S1 anterior horn cells). The tendon is lightly struck. If the reflex is not obtained, the foot is further extended and the tendon struck again. If the patient is flat in bed, the leg is externally rotated and slightly flexed at the knees. The foot is dorsiflexed and the tendon struck. If the patient is lying flat on his or her back, the examiner can obtain the reflex by just dorsiflexing the foot and striking the fingers. The gastrocnemius contraction can be seen and palpated with this technique. The primary root is S1 and the nerve is the medial popliteal from the sciatic. The reflex will be absent in disk disease at this level, but preserved in the face of a foot drop from a peroneal palsy.

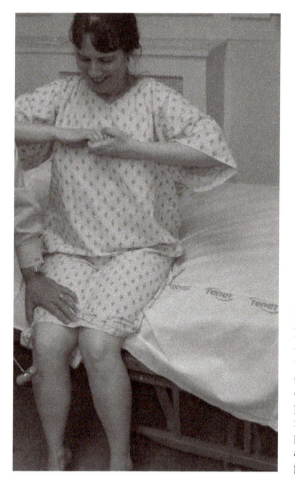

Fig. 9.4 Jendrassik's maneuver. For the upper limbs, the patient should clench the teeth tightly, or while one arm is being examined make a fist with the other. For the lower limbs, the patient interlocks the flexed fingers of the two hands and pulls one against the other and at the count of three, the patella is tapped.

Examination with reinforcement (Fig. 9.4)

Reflexes may be difficult to elicit in unrelaxed and muscular patients. Methods to increase reflex activity of the tested muscles are employed that either recruit excitatory input to the muscle by direct projections or through the reticular formation. In the upper limbs, asking the patient to make a fist on the count of three with the contralateral hand or to clench the teeth lightly will accomplish the purpose. The Jendrassik maneuver is often used for the lower extremities. The patient interlocks the flexed fingers and tries to pull them apart at the count of three when the examiner attempts to elicit the reflex.

Allied and pathologic reflexes

The Hoffman reflex (Fig. 9.5)

The fingers are dorsiflexed at the metacarpophalangeal joint and the distal phalanx flicked downwards between the examiner's index finger and thumb. Alternatively, the reflex can be obtained with the hand in the neutral position.

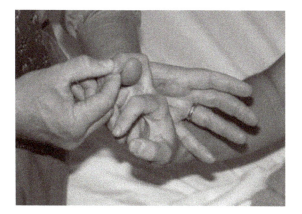

Fig. 9.5 Hoffman's sign. The terminal phalanx of the patient's middle finger is flicked downwards between the examiner's finger and thumb. In states of hyperreflexia, organic or emotional, the tips of the other fingers flex and the thumb flexes and adducts. If on one side only that is useful because this can sometimes be an early sign of unilateral pyramidal tract disease.

Analysis of the tendon reflexes

All physicians can elicit reflexes. The importance of this part of the examination is that it gives insight as to the anatomy at a segmental level and to the status of the patient's nervous system. Earlier in the chapter a brief glimpse into the physiology of reflexes was attempted prior to a discussion of the segmental and some pathologic reflexes. Reflex abnormalities are now examined by specific features.

Exaggeration

An excessively brisk reflex has a low threshold to elicit and the movement produced is sudden and short lived. If a structural lesion is present, this type of reflex usually represents upper motor neuron pathology at any level from the cortex to the anterior horn cell. It must be remembered that fright, anxiety and pain all increase reflexes through their action on the reticular activating system.

An excessively prolonged reflex occurs with cerebellar disease and hypothyroidism. Cerebellar lesions produce a pendular oscillating reflex that may take more than five oscillations before it stops. It has a large amplitude because antagonist muscles are not engaged in the normal fashion. In myxedema or general hypothyroidism, the reflex is "hung-up" because of a slow relaxation phase. This also occurs in states of protein malnutrition (a change of the elastic qualities of the tendons), hyponatremia and, rarely, syphilis.

A clonic reflex refers to continued contraction of a muscle that has been stretched once. This is most commonly seen at the ankle, knee and, rarely, the fingers. It stops when the stretch is relieved and indicates pyramidal tract disease. It may be seen in anxious individuals, particularly when extending the leg when driving. In these instances it is unsustained.

Reduction or absence of a reflex

This occurs if there is a lesion in any component of the reflex arc. This includes the sensory afferent limb (polyneuropathy, disk compression), death of the anterior horn cell (primary spinal muscular atrophy or poliomyelitis) or the ventral root (compression or GM1 antibody attack of the motor roots). The terminal nerve endings and the muscle itself may be discharging to such a degree as to block reflexes. This is exemplified by Isaac's disease (terminal twig continuous firing).

Spinal shock causes a loss of all excitatory input below the lesion with consequent loss of all reflex activity. Cerebral shock is similar, but not to the same degree. Spasticity and reflex hyperexcitability often return by 6 weeks after a cerebral insult, but occasionally within hours or days. A Babinski sign may be seen prior to the return of reflex activity.

If the patient is excessively rigid (akinetic-rigid states such as striato-nigral degeneration) or spasticity (birth injury or anoxia), the limb is splinted and a reflex may not be attainable. Ankylosed joints are unable to move, but their tendons demonstrate the expected contraction.

The superficial reflexes

The abdominal reflexes

The abdomen is lightly stroked with the back of a reflex hammer or a pencil. All four quadrants of the abdomen are lightly stroked from lateral to medial. A normal response is for the muscles of the stimulated quadrant to contract which pulls the umbilicus to that quadrant. The segmental innervations tested are:

1 epigastric T7–T9;
2 upper abdominals T9–T11;
3 lower abdominals T11–T12 (overlaps with L1).

Abnormal responses

Exaggerated abdominal reflexes are seen with anxiety. Absent abdominal reflexes occur with any lesion of the segmental reflex arc (herpes zoster or surgery) as well as with corticospinal tract lesions above the tested segment. This is more frequently seen with ipsilateral suprasegmental or contralateral pyramidal tract lesions. This finding may be intermittent. The reflex is easily fatigued so that the most accurate assessment will be the first time that it is elicited. Rarely, an inverted response occurs in which stimulation on the abnormal side (where the reflexes are absent) produces contractions of the normal side.

The abdominal reflexes are often lost early in multiple sclerosis. They may persist through late stages of the disease. They are not lost in amyotrophic lateral sclerosis (ALS) or myasthenia gravis. They may be hyperactive in corticospinal disease of long standing. This may be confirmed by a thoracoabdominal reflex in which the last rib is tapped and the umbilicus is pulled to that side.

The cremasteric reflexes

The reflex causes contraction of the dartos scroti muscle which contracts the scrotum and elevates the testicle. It is elicited by a light stroke with the back of the reflex hammer of the inner thigh. It is a segmental reflex that evaluates L1–L2. It is helpful when evaluating a patient for a high lumbar plexopathy which occurs with diabetes, lymphoma, autoimmune disease and rarely Lyme disease or periarteritis nodosa. The reflex may be lost in elderly patients with scrotal operations or hydroceles. It also is an inconstant sign of contralateral pyramidal tract disease.

The anal reflex

The perianal skin is lightly stroked with an applicator that elicits contraction of the anal sphincter. The segmental innervation is S5.

The bulbocavernosus reflex

This reflex in conjunction with the anal reflex examines the conus medullaris and the sacral spinal cord. It obviously should never be performed without a chaperone. The examiner places the third finger in the anus. The forefinger and the fourth finger then rest against the muscles of the perineum. The tip of the penis is pinched (S1 root) which causes reflex contraction of the bulbocavernosus muscle (L4–L5) as well as the external anal sphincter S4–S5. The reflex is best tested by a urologist.

The Babinski response (Fig. 9.6)

This is one of the most helpful signs in all of neurology. It demonstrates a lesion of the corticospinal tract above L1. The reflex extends from S1 to L1.

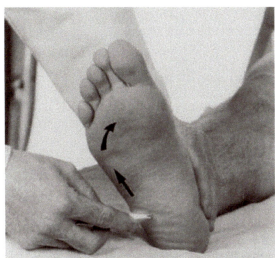

Fig. 9.6 The Babinski sign. The Babinski sign is extension of the great toe at the metatarsophalangeal joint with associated fanning of the other toes.

The very first sign of abnormality is slight contraction of the tensor fascia lata (muscle of the thigh) as the outside of the foot is stroked. The little toe abducts rather than adducting and flexing. As the stimulus progresses further up the foot, the great toe extends at the metatarsophalangeal joint in association with extension of the interphalangeal joints. The other toes abduct, fan and dorsiflex. The reflex is usually slow and unfolds in the manner described but may be jerky and repetitive. If the entire foot extends this may be voluntary. If only the great toe extends with abduction of the little toe, this is more reliable for a true Babinski sign.

Frequently, the toe will be extended prior to the reflex being attempted in severe spastic states. An extended toe is also a sign of basal ganglia disease. Toes that seem to oscillate between flexion and extension are called "intermediate" and signify corticospinal disease. If the etiology of the corticospinal dysfunction is in the spinal cord, Babinski signs are elicited prior to the hammer or key reaching the forefoot. The easier it is to elicit the response the more likely the lesion is at a spinal level. In patients with long-standing disease or those with severe lesions, the onset of the stimulus at S1 provokes dorsiflexion of the foot in association with hip and knee flexion with contraction of the tensor facia lata (a mass reflex). If the pyramidal disease is severe and long-standing, the receptive field from which the reflex can be elicited spreads from S1 to include the leg and the thigh. If the foot is amputated, a partial reflex (contraction of the tensor fascia lata) can often be attained from stimulating the stump.

Alternative plantar reflexes

These are not as reliable as the standard method of testing a plantar reflex, but may be employed in patients who will not or cannot cooperate with the examination.

The Oppenheim reflex is performed by placing the thumb and index finger on the anterior edge of the tibia and stroking downwards. More pressure is applied to the medial side of the tibia. The Gordon reflex is a hard squeeze of the gastrocnemius muscle. The Chaddock reflex is elicited by lightly stroking the lateral side of the foot below the external malleolus.

Other significant reflexes

The grasp reflex is important in both medial frontal lobe lesions and degenerative brain disease. It can be divided into the following:
1 an instinctual grasp;
2 a true grasp;
3 a traction response;
4 cross modality magnetic response.

The four components of the grasp response are related to the degree of degeneration of the motor columns of the cortex. These columns are laminated into six layers. Layers I and VI connect adjacent columns of the cortex. Layers II and III receive touch fibers and III and IV receive proprioceptive afferents. Layer V is for Betz cells and the motor efferent system. A stimulus drawn across the fifth digit to the web between the thumb and index finger stimulates C8–C6 across the motor columns of the cortex. The type of grasp response can be correlated to the level of degeneration of these cortical motor columns.

The reflex is elicited by drawing the handle of the hammer from the fourth and fifth digit across the palm. As this is performed, cortical motor columns from C8 to C6 are stimulated. If there is minimal degeneration of the columns, the patient makes several grasping movements that resemble a palpation of the object, but do not fully close the hand around the object. As degeneration proceeds and deeper layers of the motor cortical columns degenerate, the patient feels the object and then closes the hand around it which cannot be voluntarily released. This is a true grasp and is the sign that most call the "grasp response." It represents degeneration of layers II–III of the motor columns. As cortical degeneration proceeds and layers III–IV are affected, a traction response is elicited. The patient's fingers are flexed and opposed to the examiner's. The examiner pulls against the flexed fingers of the patient (stimulating deep muscle tendon and proprioceptive afferents) and the patient is unable to release the traction (Fig. 9.7). If degeneration is severe in all layers of the motor cortex and other areas of the integrated motor system, a "magnetic" response is elicited. The examiner places his or her hand slightly above the patient's and moves it. The hand of the patient is not touched, but the patient's hand follows the examiner's as if the hand was magnetized. This always signifies severe degeneration of the cortex.

The forced groping reflex or forced grasp reflex

This is a modification of the magnetic response. The examiner repeatedly touches the side of the palm and the patient attempts to grab the stimulus. This is seen with diffuse cortical degeneration.

Parietal avoidance

The patient, when approached, turns the head away from the examiner and will not allow a fundoscopic evaluation. As the examiner attempts to use the ophthalmoscope, the patient forcibly closes the eyes. If the hand is stimulated in the manner used to elicit a grasp response, the patient opens the hand and withdraws it from the examiner. These reflexes are seen with severe cortical degenerative processes with bilateral damage of the parietal lobe.

The sucking reflex

Touching the lip or corner of the mouth produces head deviation to the side of the lesion in association with a sucking movement of the lips. This is normal in infants, but is a sign of diffuse cortical degeneration in adults.

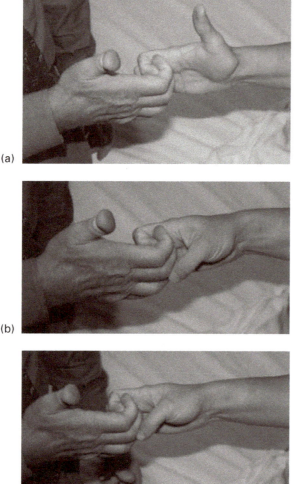

(a)

(b)

(c)

Fig. 9.7 Wartenberg's sign. The patient supinates the hand, slightly flexing the fingers. The examiner pronates his or her hand and links the similarly flexed fingers with the patient's. Both then flex their fingers further against each other's resistance. Normally, the thumb extends, although the terminal phalanx may flex slightly. In pyramidal tract lesions, the thumb adducts and flexes strongly. Unfortunately, this is not a constant sign, but if present on one side only it can indicate an early stage of pyramidal tract disease.

The palmomental reflex (Fig. 9.8)

Another degenerative or inhibited skin reflex is the palmomental response. The examiner sharply stimulates the thenar eminence and there is contralateral contraction of the mentalis muscle of the chin.

The glabellar tap (Fig. 9.9)

A normal person will blink if gently tapped on the glabella above the bridge of the nose. Blinking usually disappears after 4–5 taps. If the reflex does not accommodate it is pathologic. It is often seen early in Parkinson's disease, but may be seen in any degenerative process.

Rossolimo's reflex

The patient lies on his or her back and the ankle is slightly dorsiflexed. The ball of the foot is lightly tapped. The reflex is present when all toes contract.

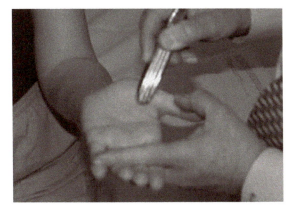

Fig. 9.8 The palmomental reflex. The edge of a reflex hammer is lightly stroked from medial to lateral across the thenar eminence. This causes ipsilateral contraction of the mentalis muscle of the chin. This reflex is encountered in severe degenerative brain disease.

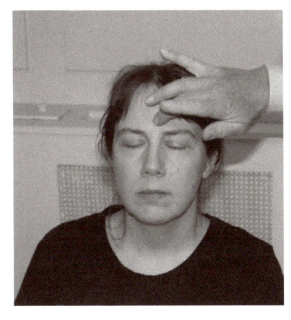

Fig. 9.9 The glabellar tap. A normal person can inhibit blinking within 4–5 taps of the bridge of the nose. A patient with a positive Meyerson's sign or glabellar reflex has synchronous blinking after 5 taps. This sign is most often seen with Parkinson's disease or diffuse organic brain disease.

Flexion of all toes can also be accomplished by the same maneuver as is used in a Hoffman's reflex, in this instance utilizing the middle toe. If positive, the reflex demonstrates disinhibition of the spinal cord from a higher lesion.

The corneal mandibular reflex

In an unconscious patient, stimulation of the cornea may elicit contralateral deviation of the jaw. This signifies disinhibition of the fifth nerve motor nucleus and a structural lesion above the mid pons.

The classic signs

Chvostek's sign

This is a sign that denotes partial depolarization of the facial nerve, usually from a low ionized calcium level. The examiner taps over the entrance of the facial nerve as it exits the parotid gland which produces twitching and retraction of the corner of the mouth. It is also rarely seen with regeneration of a damaged facial nerve or with motor neuron disease.

Trousseau's sign

This is a flexion contracture of the hand and wrist produced by slight ischemia or nerve irritability from application of a sphygmomanometer. This also denotes latent tetany and can be accelerated and increased by hyperventilation.

Lhermitte's sign

Flexing the neck forward causes shock-like sensations down the arms, legs or spine. It may be seen only in the lower limbs or contralaterally. It is thought to occur from irritation of the dorsal columns. The spinal cord and nerve roots move (1.5 cm) with flexion of the neck. It is most commonly seen in patients with multiple sclerosis, but also is noted with cervical spondylosis, vitamin B_{12} deficiency, Chiari malformations and irradiation myelopathy.

10: Coordination

Smooth movements require modulation during all of their component parts. A movement has to be planned and then executed. Planning of movements occurs in the prefrontal and supplementary motor cortex as well as the posterior parietal lobe and is reflected electrically by a cortical negative potential. The patient must have a general knowledge of the expected results of the movement which are then matched with the actual result (efferent copy). It is convenient to divide movements into thirds so that initiation, feed forward, feed back and terminal components can be analyzed. As a movement is initiated, the first third has a great deal to do with its planning (praxis) and the modulation is due to feed forward mechanisms from collateral fibers leaving the corticospinal tracts and synapsing in the thalamus which are then projected back to the primary sensory cortex which can effect early components of the motor output. The middle third of a movement is modulated from collaterals of the motor output that synapse with the dorsal column nuclei that in turn project to the thalamus and primary sensory cortex. Proprioceptive feedback from the displaced joints to the cerebellar intermediate zone projects to the ventrointermediate (VIM) nucleus of the thalamus. Movement requires planning, initiation and maintenance as well as integrated feed forward and feed back mechanisms to remain correctly online. In addition, it requires the proper moderation of agonists and antagonists so that there is no difficulty with its termination or timing. The parietal lobe is required to anchor the patient in space and compare the posture to where it should be in space (the subjective visual vertical). The limbic system and its motor loops determine specific movements under stress and control the desire to move. It is clear that a great deal of the human nervous system is required to initiate, maintain and complete a simple smooth movement.

Most clinical testing of coordination is aimed at assessing the function of the cerebellum that modulates movement from proprioceptive feedback.

The major function of the cerebellum is to coordinate:

1   agonists and antagonist muscles at each joint;
2   to smooth the termination of a movement;
3   to energize movements along with the sustaining input from the outflow of the basal ganglia.

It has been recently shown that in addition to its role in movement, the cerebellum has a major function in cognition.

The upper limb

Preliminary observations

A broad-based gait, scanning speech with poor articulation and hypometric eye movements have all been noted prior to testing the extremities during the earlier parts of the examination (i.e., during the history and walk to the examining room). The major tests of the cerebellum are to evaluate its ability to smoothly control agonist and antagonist muscles.

A cerebellar drift is upward with the eyes closed and the arms outstretched. There is abnormal overcontracture of the flexors of the hand at the metacarpophalangeal and proximal interphalangeal joints which cause a "spooned" hand posture.

The examiner lightly taps the outstretched arm to displace it downward. The examiner watches for the abnormality or overshoot as the patient attempts to place the arm in its former position. This maneuver should be performed with the eyes open and then closed. If the patient performs well with the eyes open and not closed, there is visual compensation for a proprioceptive deficit. The patient is then asked to close the eyes and the arm is pressed downwards against resistance and suddenly released. A normal person controls the displacement very well as there is normal braking of the movement with little displacement. Another means of evaluating both pyramidal and cerebellar control of fine movement is asking the patient to tap the thumb and index finger, repetitively. The examiner evaluates the amplitude of each movement and the facility with which it is accomplished. This aspect of movement can further be evaluated by having the patient tap all other fingers to the thumb. In cerebellar disease the amplitude and rhythm vary. In pyramidal disease the movements have normal rhythm but are not fractioned and have poor facility.

Abnormalities of cerebellar function (Fig. 10.1)

When the patient is first asked to raise the arm to evaluate a drift, a patient with isolated cerebellar disease will overshoot on the affected side and then with visual compensation move the abnormal arm to be parallel with the normal side. The arm may have several oscillations and tends to deviate to the normal side. A cerebellar drift is upwards on the affected side with partial wrist flexion and extension of the metacarpophalangeal and proximal interphalangeal joints (spooning). If the arm drifts sideways this may be a postural deficit, which is also seen with cervical cord lesions as proprioception of the arm is controlled by the cuneocerebellar pathways of the cervical cord. Polyminimyoclonus, unusual posture of the fingers and external rotation of the hand, may be noted in dystonia and proprioceptive deficits from parietal lesions. Thalamic proprioceptive loss is accompanied by a thalamic hand and severe proprioceptive loss from dorsal column involvement is often associated with flailing arm movements.

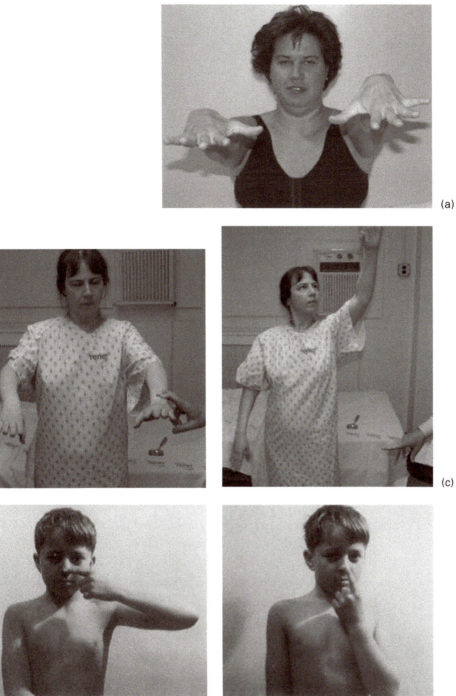

Fig. 10.1 (a) Cerebellar drift. The hand and arm drift upward on extension. Note the uneven interplay between agonist and antagonist flexors and extensor hand muscles. This causes "spooning" of the hand. (b) Overshoot. The examiner presses down on the patient's arm and asks that the patient maintain it at its original position. (c) The patient is unable to brake the agonist muscle and cannot keep the arm at the original position – it overshoots upwards. (d) Classic finger–nose–finger test. (*Cont'd on page 210*).

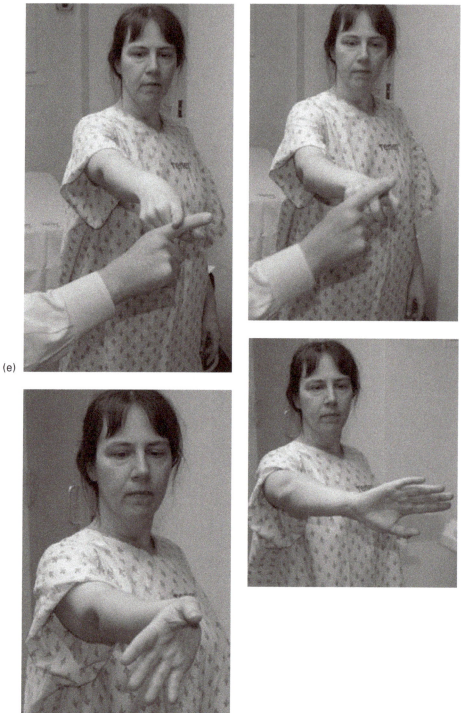

(e)

(f)

(g)

(h)

Fig. 10.1 (*cont'd*) (e) The patient is asked to touch the moving finger with hers. Note: she misses dorsally. (f) Ventrally, she is also past-pointing and slides past the target. (g) Dysdiadochokinesis. The patient is asked to alternatively pronate and supinate her arm. Each rotation is observed and the patient with cerebellar disease slips past the expected end-point and produces a series of non-facile wide amplitude movements. Thumb up. (h) Thumb down.

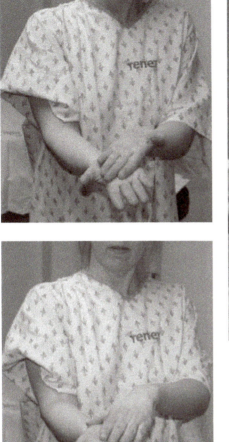

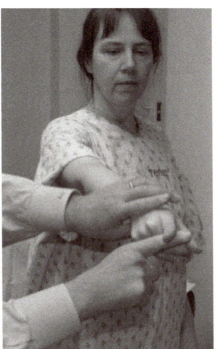

(i)

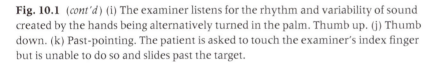

(j)

(k)

Fig. 10.1 (*cont'd*) (i) The examiner listens for the rhythm and variability of sound created by the hands being alternatively turned in the palm. Thumb up. (j) Thumb down. (k) Past-pointing. The patient is asked to touch the examiner's index finger but is unable to do so and slides past the target.

Abnormal displacement and rebound of the patient's arm with the eyes closed after tapping may be caused by the following:

1 weakness where it remains in the displaced position;

2 cerebellar hypotonia where it oscillates after being displaced;

3 severe proprioceptive deficits in which the patient does not realize the new position and misplaces the arm.

Cerebellar disease manifests as a problem with proper timing of agonist and antagonist muscle interaction. This is most easily shown by manifestations of the check response. The arm is displaced downward and the patient is asked to bring it to a parallel position with the normal arm. When released it overshoots the intended position and oscillates 2–3 times before this goal is attained. The problem is failure to recruit antagonist muscles quickly. This deficiency can be corrected by vision with proprioceptive deficits. Patients with proprioceptive deficits (eyes closed) leave the hand and arm in the displaced position but, with vision restored, recorrect inaccurately without oscillating.

Finger tapping, particularly when the index finger is apposed to the crease of the distal interphalangeal joint, is an excellent screen for function of the major components of the motor system. In pyramidal disease, the fingers tend to move in concert (failure to fractionalize movement) and tapping fatigues. Extrapyramidal disease is suspected when it is difficult for the patient to initiate and sustain movement. The latter is best exemplified by a Parkinson's disease patient's handwriting. It gets progressively smaller to become illegible by the end of the sentence. In cerebellar disease, each movement is different from its predecessor. There are wide amplitude swings. The proximal wrist joint is not fixed; the table (proximal wrist) is not steady for the fine pyramidal movements required. Chorea is characterized by the intrusion of both proximal and distal movements that destroy the motor pattern. In dystonia, the patient may have proximal muscle overflow (the patient cannot restrict the pattern of muscles recruited) or cannot break a distal abnormally held posture.

The finger–nose–finger test (see Fig. 10.1c)

The patient is asked to touch the nose with the forefinger after the arm is abducted and to lightly hold the finger in this position. The examiner observes the smoothness of the movements, the accuracy of the placement and the ability to hold the finger in its new position. The test is repeated with the eyes closed. A further amplification of the test is asking the patients to touch the examiner's forefinger with their own and then to touch their own nose. The examiner makes this more challenging by moving his or her finger to new positions.

Cerebellar deficits of the ipsilateral side produce wide oscillation in the terminal one-third of movement and then gradually the side-to-side oscillations dampen. There is a slight tendency to overshoot the object to the side of the lesion. The side-to-side wavering is different from an intention tremor which increases during the last third of movement when the target is approached (rubral tremor).

A postural kinetic tremor occurs when the patient is asked to hold the arms in front of the chest with spread fingers opposed. This maneuver induces vertical oscillations. This tremor results from interruption of the dentate nuclear outflow to the thalamic cerebellar area. The larger the oscillations the closer the lesion is to the red nucleus. This is called a "rubral tremor" although the red nucleus is not involved. The oscillations are at right angles to the line of movement and often increase as the target is approached.

The lower limb

The same maneuvers that are used for the arm are used for the leg with the realization that much less dexterity is expected. The patient is asked to touch the examiner's fingers with his or her great toe. This is easily accomplished in a normal person with minimal terminal oscillation. Tapping of the foot should be rhythmic. The examiner watches for amplitude and arrhythmia of the movement.

The heel–knee test

The patient is asked to place the foot on the opposite knee and to move it up and down. Care must be taken to have the patient balance the heel on the tibia and not perform the movement with the heel on the side of the tibia. The movement is performed with the eyes closed. The patient is asked to tap on the heel on the opposite knee where rhythm and amplitude can be easily observed.

In severe cerebellar disease, the heel overshoots the tibia laterally with a rotary oscillation which is equivalent to the intention tremor noted in the arm. The movement is completed with side-to-side oscillations and ends on the dorsum of the foot in an uncontrolled manner.

In proprioceptive or sensory ataxia (dorsal column, large fiber neuropathy or dorsal root ganglia disease), the patient is unaware of the position of the heel to the knee and lifts it too high prior to the start of the test. The deficits noted are not oscillatory. The heel may fall off the tibia several times during the maneuver and the patient will only be able to try again by placing the heel on the thigh and sliding it down to touch the knee. In patients with cerebellar and posterior column disease, elements of both deficits are present. The movement is poor with or without visual compensation.

Dysdiadochokinesis (see Fig. 10.1g–j)

This is failure of agonist–antagonist muscle function that is clinically manifest as inability to perform rapid alternating movements. The patient is asked to extend the arms and rotate them back and forth rapidly at the wrists. Patients with cerebellar disease slide past the end-point with each rotation so that the movement is coarse, irregular and slow. If the patient clenches the fist and attempts the rotation, a jerky flexion extension movement is superimposed on the rotation.

Past-pointing tests (see Fig. 10.1k)

The examiner asks the patient to rapidly touch the examiner's forefinger with the their own. The patient is unable to brake the movement as it nears the examiner's and the finger slides past the end-point (failure to engage the antagonist muscles correctly). Another way to check this function is to have the patient hold the arms horizontally opposed to the examiner and then asked to raise them above the horizontal and return to their original position with the eyes open and then closed. In cerebellar disease, the arm deviates toward the side of the lesion as well as upwards. In labyrinthine disease, both arms will deviate towards the side of the lesion, which is the same deviation as the slow component of the nystagmus (the fast cortical component will be to the opposite side).

Rapid hand tapping (see Fig. 10.1i,j)

The examiner listens to the tap of one hand on the back of the other. In cerebellar disease, the taps are irregular and of different amplitude. The tap may also develop a rotary stroking movement. This is further exacerbated by having the patient alternate taps on the palms and dorsal surfaces of the hand. Listening to the tap of the foot with the heel down is effective in the lower extremity.

Tapping in a circle

The patient is asked to hit a target within a circle with a pencil. The dots will be scattered over a wide area in any form of ataxia, but will be more prominent to the side of an ipsilateral cerebellar lesion.

Spiral drawing

The patient is asked to draw a spiral. In cerebellar disease, it will become progressively large and irregular. The same occurs with handwriting.

11: Disorders of Speech

The ability to make and understand language is uniquely human and defects are categorized as aphasia. These extend to reading and writing. Although advances have been made with magnetic resonance imaging (MRI), functional MRI, single photon emission computed tomography (SPECT) and positron emission tomography (PET) scanning, all we can currently accomplish is to localize speech deficits. Until we can understand how inanimate material, lipids, membranes, sodium-potassium ATPase and the structure of the brain can become sensate we will not understand behavioral neurology (Aristotle's "mind–brain barrier").

Dysarthria refers to articulation of the spoken word. It requires excellent tongue movement against the teeth (glottals), precise movement of the mouth and lips (labials), closing of the nasopharynx (tensor veli palatini) and the coordination of speech and breathing.

A conscious patient who makes no attempt to speak or make a sound is mute. An akinetic mute patient does not speak, is paralyzed, but may reflexly follow the examiner with the eyes. An abulic patient proffers nothing and may only respond with a yes or no answer to intense stimulation. This is often the result of a subfrontal lesion. Amazingly, if handed a toy telephone, the patient may speak into it. Mutism, in general, is caused by lesions of the anterior wall of the third ventricle and bilateral lesions of the posterior medial frontal lobes as well as subfrontal lesions (anterior communicating aneurysm or head trauma; rarely a tumor). Total mutism may occur from a stem middle cerebral artery (MCA) embolus or supplementary motor area lesion (SMA supplementary area of the frontal lobe). Most often under these conditions the patient appears stunned, but occasionally gives the impression of trying to speak, but is unable to produce words. An aphonic patient is able to speak, but cannot produce any words or has a greatly diminished volume. This type of aphonia is caused by disease of the larynx or vocal cords. If the patient has a normal cough, this is hysterical. Disorders of voice volume from central lesions most often are secondary to disease of the basal ganglia (Parkinson's disease or of the cortex, cerebral hypophonia).

Dysarthria

The ability to speak clearly requires bilateral coordination of the tongue, lips, palate, larynx and respiration. Almost all levels of the neuraxis are involved. Each level of involvement can usually be discerned. The most severe articulation problems come from lesions of the frontal operculum and the brainstem nuclei. The frontal operculum is the cortical center for the muscles of articulation and breathing. Bilateral lesions, usually occurring from severe head trauma or seriatim MCA strokes cause aphemia. This is a gutteral dysarthria so severe that it does not sound like human speech. Lesions of the centrum semiovale, the anterior limb of the internal capsule, and the posterior ventral third of the pons all cause dysarthria. Rarely, lesions of the medulla, affecting the twelfth nerve in particular, cause severe dysarthria. Lesions of the basal ganglia cause severe hypophonia. The patient may produce an explosive onset of speech after a long period when attempting to speak. Cerebellar speech has a scanning quality in which the patient has difficulty coordinating breathing and speaking. amyotrophic lateral sclerosis (ALS) patients have severe dysarthria resulting from weakness and atrophy of all bulbar musculature.

Examination of dysarthria

The examiner should have a good idea of the patient's articulation abilities from taking the history. Ask the patient to enunciate "British artillery brigade" and distinguish whether he or she has more trouble with labials ("British") or glottals ("artillery") where the tongue is pressed against the lips. The examiner should have a clear picture of the loudness, rhythm, modulation and tone of speech (partial deafness or weakness of the tensor veli palatini cause nasal tone) as well as the constancy of the deficit.

Spastic dysarthria

This is usually caused by bilateral upper motor neuron disease or lesions of the corticospinal tract, which occur with motor neuron disease, head trauma, upper brainstem tumors and all causes of pseudobulbar palsy. In this condition, the tongue is small, the speech spastic and there is limited movement of the lips and mouth. Patients have particular difficulty with the letters "b," "p," "d" and "r". The patient appears to be speaking from the back of the throat. There is usually associated spasticity, a Babinski sign and increased jaw and pharyngeal reflexes. At times, there is an explosive quality to speech as it is initiated.

Extrapyramidal dysarthria

The speech is hypophonic and monotonous. Inflection and modulation are lost, words run into one another and sentences start and stop suddenly. There is associated hypomimia (lack of facial expression and decreased movement of the tongue and lips). The ends of a sentence may be spoken explosively and palilalia is common (the constant repetition of a particular syllable).

Ataxic dysarthria

The difficulty in this instance is with the coordination of the muscles of speech and breathing. The patient's speech is irregular, slurred, changes from loud to soft, and is arrhythmic. The words merge one with another or are spaced incorrectly. The speech may have a staccato or explosive quality and this is incoordination of speech with breathing (scanning). The usual causes are all forms of hereditary cerebellar disease, multiple sclerosis, drug intoxications, superior cerebellar artery stroke and tumors.

Dysarthria resulting from lesions of lower motor neurons and muscles

Individual words or sounds are poorly articulated depending on the level of involvement. Facial paralysis makes it difficult to pronounce labials such as "b," "p," "m" or "w". Tongue weakness and paralysis causes severe dysarthria in all spheres. Words with "l," "d," "n," "s," "t," "x" and "z" are particularly difficult. Palatal paralysis or weakness produces nasal speech because of weakness of the tensor veli palatini. The letters "b" and "d" sound like "m", while "n" and "g" are distorted to "rh", "k" sounds like "na." The patient's speech becomes worse when the head is bent forward.

Myasthenic dysarthria

The voice may be normal with rest or at the beginning of each sentence, but changes as speech progresses. Palatal weakness and hoarseness occur.

Aphasia

Aphasia is the loss or impairment of language function caused by structural or functional brain damage. The latter refers to seizure activity, transient ischemia, abnormal electrolyte, endocrine or toxic states.

Aphasia encompasses deficits in the following:
1 prosody, the rhythm of speech;
2 timbre, speech modulation;
3 naming (small parts of common objects);
4 the ability to follow commands off the midline;
5 repetition of individual words or a sentence;
6 reading and writing;
7 color naming.

Preliminary information

Prior to testing a patient for aphasia, the examiner needs to determine the patient's native language, education level, prior ability to read, write,

217

spell, calculate and handedness. Most right-handed patients are strongly dominant for language in the left hemisphere. This is true approximately 99% of the time. Left-handed individuals are 90% dominant for language in the left hemisphere. They have mixed dominance and in general do better with language recovery after damage to the dominant hemisphere. Up until the age of 6 years, a brain injury to the dominant hemisphere can be overcome as speech mechanisms switch to the contralateral hemisphere.

Spontaneous speech

The aphasia examination starts by the examiner listening to the quality and quantity of spontaneous speech. Anterior speech areas, Broca's area and the SMA initiate and maintain expressive speech. Wernicke's area (21/22, the posterior third of the dominant temporal lobe) decodes speech. No aphasia is pure; all have elements of expressive and receptive deficits. Difficulty with prosody and fluency argue strongly for an anterior aphasia while normal fluency and prosody is characteristic of a posterior aphasia. Anterior aphasias are accompanied by hemiparesis and subtle ideomotor apraxias as well as agrammatisms. Posterior aphasias have a pressure of speech, the rhythm and prosody are normal, but speech is often contaminated by translittoral aphasic errors (two consonants used together), word substitutions (green for red) and neologisms ("garunch" for garage). The patient often uses a long sentence to describe a noun to overcome failure to find the correct word ("it is used to write" for "pen").

Comprehension

Patients can utilize both hemispheres to perform midline commands such as "Stick your tongue out," "Get up" and "Close your eyes." Comprehension needs to be tested by commands that are off the midline. Severely affected patients should be able to answer simple questions with a yes or no ("Is it a sunny day?"). A patient is asked to point up or down with the thumb or to point out objects in the room. The patient may then be asked to place specific objects in specific places.

Naming objects

All aphasias have a degree of nominal aphasia. Lesions of the supramarginal gyrus may give a rather pure nominal aphasia. The patient is asked to name small parts of common objects such as a watch or pen. The examiner notes the speed of the patient's response, paraphasias, neologisms and perseveration. A patient who names small parts of common objects quickly and correctly is not aphasic. The test can be sharpened by asking the patient to pick out objects in front of him or her by name.

Repetition

The patient is asked to repeat a simple sentence and then a complex word. This test evaluates Wernicke's area (decodes language), the arcuate fasciculus that connects Wernicke's and Broca's areas which initiates expressive speech. Patients with a conduction aphasia, a disconnection between Broca's and Wernicke's areas, often do better with a complicated word than a simple one. If asked to repeat "Today is a sunny day," they may be hesitant and stammer "Today sunny." They may easily enunciate "presidential address."

Reading

The posterior parietal areas 39–41 as well as Wernicke's area are critically important for reading and decoding language. The patient is asked to read individual words, sentences and then instructions to perform specific actions.

Writing

Errors in grammar are most characteristic of anterior aphasias. All posterior aphasic patients have writing disabilities. Exner's area, immediately anterior to Broca's area, in addition to Wernicke's and areas 39–41 seems to be important for writing. If this area is damaged, patient's have more difficulty writing than their degree of weakness would suggest. Patients are asked to write their name and address, to take dictation and to write a few sentences about the weather.

Calculation

This is not strictly a part of the examination for aphasia, but is important as a component of posterior aphasia pathology and particularly von Gerstmann's syndrome. Dyscalculia is frequently seen with posterior parietal deficits.

Anatomic points regarding aphasia

The major speech areas are located pre- or postsylvian fissure. If a lesion is anterior or posterior perisylvian, the ability to repeat is often involved. In general, if a patient who is aphasic repeats well, there is no perisylvian pathology. These aphasias (lesions around the primary speech areas) are noted as transcortical. Lesions that produce a transcortical motor aphasia are superior to Broca's area and have many of its features. A transcortical sensory aphasia occurs from lesions posterior and inferior to Wernicke's area. These aphasias frequently occur in watershed distributions between anterior cerebral artery (ACA)/MCA anteriorly and MCA/posterior cerebral artery (PCA) posteriorly from cerebral hypotension and ischemia (stroke, anoxia and cardiac surgery). If Wernicke's and Broca's areas are spared as well as the arcuate fasciculus, speech areas are isolated from the rest of the brain and an isolation of the speech area aphasia occurs. These patients proffer nothing spontaneously, understand poorly but are able to repeat. This type of aphasia occurs with hypotension and carbon monoxide poisoning. It is rare.

Broca's aphasia

The major components of Broca's aphasia are difficulty initiating and articulating speech, non-fluency and an output of less than 20 words per minute. The phrases are short, have abnormal prosody, inflection and timbre. Substantive words are used without syntactic language. There is decreased use of articles, and grammatic modifiers. These patients have a specific defect in use of syntactic aspects of language. Repetition is abnormal, particularly for simple syntactic words and endings. Comprehension is deficient, often for syntactic function words such as the difference between "in" and "on." Confrontation naming is poor, but can be improved with phonetic or contextual cues. Reading comprehension is poor because of failure to comprehend grammatically significant words. Writing is difficult out of proportion to the degree of weakness. There are omissions of grammatic words and misspelling of substantive words. A significant number of patients have an apraxia of handling objects and initiation of movement with the left arm and face (if the patient is left hemisphere dominant).

Wernicke's aphasia

These patients have normal prosody and phrase length, often with a normal to increased rate of word production. Grammatic structure is nearly normal although there are few substantive words. Language is dominated by literal or phonemic paraphasic errors, consonant errors, neologisms, circumlocution and word substitutions. These patients cannot comprehend or repeat spoken language. Naming of small common objects is impaired. Reading and writing is involved to a varying degree. Some patients are "word deaf" (they can understand other sounds) while others are "word blind" (cannot read words, but do recognize other objects). Many patients early on are unaware of their deficit and do not understand why others cannot comprehend their speech. There is no hemiparesis, but patients may have a superior quadrantic visual field defect. Apraxia on imitation of object handling may be present.

Conduction aphasia

These defects are caused by defects in the arcuate fasciculus. Patients are usually fluent. Their comprehension is better preserved than their ability to repeat. Naming is deficient because of literal paraphasic substitutions.

Reading aloud is poor, but comprehension is relatively well preserved. There are omissions, spelling errors and altered word sequences of words and letters in the patient's written output. Most lesions producing conduction aphasia are in the supramarginal gyrus or arcuate fasciculus.

Transcortical motor aphasia

Patients have difficulty in initiating speech. They stammer and stutter, but repeat sentences easily. They have more difficulty naming than with comprehension. Writing is poor but they can read aloud and comprehend well. They often have a hemiparesis and apraxia of the left hand to command (decoded in Wernicke's area), but an engram of the movement is encoded in the left premotor area which has to be transmitted across the midline and activate the contralateral primary motor cortex. Lesions that cause a transcortical motor aphasia (TCM) aphasia are in the supplementary motor area or high in the dorsolateral prefrontal cortex above Broca's area.

Global aphasia

These patients have lesions in both frontal and parietotemporal cortex. The usual lesion is a carotid occlusion with an isolated hemisphere (poor cross-filling from the contralateral side due to atretic anterior and posterior communicating arteries) or a stem MCA occlusion. Rarely, a superior division MCA artery occlusion causes this pattern which soon evolves into a Broca's aphasia. These patients cannot initiate speech, read, write, follow commands, repeat or name. Most have a concomitant right hemiparesis.

Anomic aphasia

This is the most common aphasia and is a component of all aphasias. Patients are unable to find the correct word in spontaneous speech, writing or on confrontation. Their prosody is normal as is repetition and comprehension. Patients may find words more easily while writing than with spontaneous speech.

There are usually concomitant deficits which may be subtle in comprehension and writing. A variety of lesions have been described for this type of aphasia which include the left temporoparietal junction, frontal, temporal and parietal lobes. A supramarginal gyrus lesion may give a relatively pure anomic aphasia. Brain tumors have been reported to give a slowly progressive anomic aphasia. It is frequently recorded in neurodegenerative disease, post head injury and with metabolic and toxic disorders.

Subcortical aphasia

These types of aphasia have not been completely characterized. They have been described with lesions of the AV and DM nuclei of the thalamus and

221

the caudate and putamen nuclei of the basal ganglia. They may have an acute onset with initial mutism and resemble more of a Broca's than Wernicke's profile. The verbal output is slow and poorly articulated, spastic dysarthric and abnormalities of pitch have been noted. Reduplicative speech, in which the patient repeats the last components of words and sentences, has been seen. Some patients have concomitant hyperkinetic and slurred speech. Naming and reading are relatively well preserved.

Aphemia

This is a most severe form of dysarthria. The lesion destroys the frontal operculum, which is the cortical motor innervation for the tenth, twelfth and seventh nerve. These patients are so dysarthric as to be unintelligible. They can fully comprehend written and spoken language. Word choice and syntax are normal. They are often mute at onset. A unilateral lesion that causes aphemia is in Broca's area or undercuts the white matter of the left frontal operculum. As the patient recovers, he or she has cerebral hypophonia and severely dysrhythmic speech. Prosody is similar to an anterior aphasia, but is grammatically intact. Lesions of the anterior cingulate gyrus, the medial frontal cortex and the supplementary motor cortex may simulate aphasia.

Stuttering and stammering

Recent evidence points to structural lesions in speech output areas. The psychiatric problems are a consequence of the speech deficits.

Echolalia

Lesions of the dominant temporoparietal cortex cause this deficit. Patients involuntarily repeat words and phrases they have just heard without understanding their meaning.

Pure word articulation failure

This is an apractic rare speech problem. The patient may be totally unable to articulate a word or just have slight slurred speech. These patients can read, write and copy. Other branchial functions are normal. It is most often caused by a lesion of the left frontal operculum or hemisphere.

Pure word deafness

These patients cannot comprehend spoken language, but can identify nonverbal sound. They are fluent, can read and write, but cannot comprehend spoken language or repeat it. The anatomic lesions reported are damage to

Heschl's gyrus and destruction of the radiations from the medial geniculate body as well as callosal fibers from the contralateral superior temporal gyrus. This combination of lesions isolate the left hemisphere auditory association cortex from any auditory input. It may also be produced by bilateral damage of the mid portion of the superior temporal gyrus.

Non-verbal auditory agnosia is the inability to recognize non-verbal sounds and may occur with lesions of the right hemisphere. Cortical deafness requires bilateral damage to Heschl's gyrus and its connections. Patients are aware of words and sounds, but cannot interpret them.

Developmental auditory imperception

This is a hereditary disturbance primarily of young boys with normal hearing. They attract parental attention as they pay no attention to spoken words. They may develop their own speech as do congenitally deaf patients.

Alexia

These patients are unable to comprehend written material. They can recognize words spelled aloud, written on the palm or palpated. A few colors can usually be recognized. They are often associated with impaired naming and understanding of color names with normal color vision. There is often a nominal aphasia. The usual etiology is occlusion of the left PCA that infarcts the left occipital lobe and the splenium of the corpus callosum. This prevents transfer of word visual information to the left angular gyrus.

Alexia with agraphia (visual asymbolia) is more common than alexia without agraphia. These patients cannot read or write (with either hand) but may be able to copy with difficulty. The usual lesion is the left angular branch of the superior division of the MCA. It may be accompanied by acalculia, nominal aphasia, hemianopia and some degree of visual agnosia.

Agraphia

In general, patients who have aphasia in spoken language have abnormal writing. Agraphia is most often seen with anterior frontal (Exner's area 45) or posterior parietotemporal syndromes. The agraphia associated with Broca's aphasia is associated with large, poorly constructed words replete with misspelling and omission of function words and endings.

The agraphia of dominant posterior parietal lesions demonstrates well-formed words in abnormal sentences characterized by abnormal word order, omissions that are devoid of meaning and misspellings. Posterior parietotemporal lesions may produce agraphia with characteristic anterior type symptomatology.

Syndromes of calculating impairment

Aphasic acalculia

The patient cannot comprehend well enough to write numbers correctly or substitute one number for another. Aphasic acalculia is most often seen with lesions of the posterior parietal cortex of the speech dominant hemisphere.

Visuospatial acalculia

The patient can compute normally, but is unable to place numbers in the correct position in space. The patient can manipulate individual mathematical functions. The causative lesion is at the parietooccipital junction of the non-dominant hemisphere.

Von Gerstmann's syndrome

This is a constellation of finger agnosia, acalculia, inability to cross the midline and right–left confusion. Agraphia and a conduction aphasia, as well as constructional apraxia are also often present. More extensive involvement, which includes the angular gyrus, causes an inability to read and write as well as a nominal aphasia. The angular gyrus syndrome is von Gerstmann's syndrome, central alexia and anomic aphasia. Posterior aphasias are common with von Gerstmann's syndrome, but are not invariant.

12: Apraxias

Apraxias are the inability to perform an individual or sequential function in the face of intact motor, sensory and coordinative abilities. A specific motor function is first conceived and is denoted as an engram of movement. This finds a correlate in the cortical negative variant or Bëreitschaft (readiness) potential recorded over the prefrontal and supplementary motor cortices. This then is translated into the required movement. Disorganization of unitary or sequential engrams are the core of apraxia. Different areas of the brain when damaged cause specific apraxias.

Methods of testing

The examiner must be certain that the patient has no deficits of strength sensation or coordination that would interfere with his or her ability to perform the required tasks. The examiner asks the patient to perform a series of tasks to test specific forms of apraxia. The major apraxias tested are the following:
1 visual;
2 oral buccal lingual;
3 gait;
4 ideomotor;
5 ideational;
6 constructional;
7 callosal.

Visual praxis

The patient is asked to copy the position of the examiner's hand (Fig. 2.1). The examiner demonstrates the posture to be copied and then withdraws the hand. The patient must be able to see the requested hand position, hear and understand the task, and then form the motor program to perform it. The latter requires the patient to form an "engram" of the desired movement and then relay this to the primary motor cortex. Lesions in the prefrontal cortex and supplementary motor areas preclude the patient from making the engram and he or she will make a fist or place the fingers in an incorrect position.

Oral buccal lingual apraxia

The patient is asked to touch a tongue blade with the tongue and to touch it above the horizontal. It is striking that most patients with this form of apraxia are unable to lift their tongue above the horizontal to touch the blade. They have difficulty moving the tongue side-to-side outside of the mouth or to touch the tongue blade as requested. This often reflects degeneration of the frontal operculum which is the cortical region for all activities requiring cranial nerves involved with tongue movements, swallowing and breathing. Coughing, sneezing and involuntary movements are preserved.

Gait apraxia

The patient may have two forms of gait apraxia. The first is a "magnetic gait" in which the foot seems to be stuck to the floor and the patient can only move a few inches before it becomes stuck again. This appears to be a foot grasp. "Egg-walking" is striking. The patient gently picks the feet up as if walking on eggs, but does not advance. These gaits are caused by failure to activate various brainstem locomotor centers, particularly the nucleus cuneiformis of the midbrain. In clinical practice, it is most commonly seen with normal pressure hydrocephalus in which the descending motor fibers to the legs are closest to the dilating lateral ventricles and are compromised. These gaits are frequently seen in patients with degenerative processes and lacunar strokes that affect the descending corticospinal pathways as well as basal ganglion diseases.

Ideomotor apraxia

This form of apraxia refers to the inability of a patient to carry out a single purposeful movement such as a salute or to demonstrate how to turn a key in a lock or to comb one's hair. Patients understand the task and are able to formulate how it should be performed, but cannot perform it on command. Patients often substitute a body part for the object, such as using the index finger as a comb rather than demonstrating how to hold a comb. Patients may perform better with an object (transitive) than without (intransitive). Ideomotor apraxias may be seen with conductive aphasias. Limb-kinetic apraxia is a judgment call. The patient has a certain clumsiness when performing a simple task that is out of proportion to his or her weakness. The lack of ability to form an engram prevents the patient from imitating an act that utilizes objects.

Ideational apraxia

The patient is unable to correctly carry out the sequence of a common task although each of its component parts can be successfully performed. If given a package of cigarettes and a matchbox and asked how he or she would light a cigarette and smoke it, the patient could remove the cigarette from the package, but would strike the match against the package and fail to put the cigarette in the mouth. Lesions causing ideational apraxia are primarily in the posterior parietal areas 5 and 7. Patients may have an inability to handle real objects even though they can mimic the use of an object (the opposite of ideomotor apraxia).

Constructional apraxia

This is the inability of a patient to construct or copy a visually presented object with blocks or by drawing. The examiner may utilize four matches to construct a box and then ask the patient to copy the construction. The angles are not placed correctly and often the heads of the matches do not correspond to the examiner's construct.

The examiner must be sure that the patient can perceive the elements of the object, their spatial relationships and has the strength and coordination to perform the task. Left and right parietal lesions may cause a constructional apraxia. Right-sided lesions are more commonly associated with constructional apraxia than left and are often associated with some degree of neglect of the left side. Patients with left parietal lesions and constructional apraxia may have a concomitant fluent aphasia. A deficit of visual constructive ability is hard evidence of a parietal lesion. The supramarginal gyrus projections to the motor cortex are affected.

Callosal apraxia

Patients with callosal apraxia are unable to perform a simple task on command with the left hand. To perform a task with the left hand the patient must hear and understand the test which is accomplished by Wernicke's area (posterior one-third of the superior temporal gyrus). The information must cross the midline anteriorly in the corpus callosum to synapse in the right prefrontal area which in turn relays the information to the right primary motor cortex for execution. Lesions of both prefrontal cortices and the anterior corpus callosum can interrupt this distributed system and cause inability to utilize the left hand on command. The usual lesions that cause this deficit are prefrontal branch occlusions of the superior division of the middle cerebral artery, strokes of the anterior cerebral artery, callosotomy for epilepsy and frontal lobe gliomas.

Apraxia of eyelid opening

Patients are unable to open their eyes to command. They frequently tape the lids to their glasses. They often think they are blind but pain and startle responses open their eyes. The lesion is in the second frontal convolution of the frontal eye fields.

Dressing apraxia

The patient has inordinate difficulty in dressing or undressing themselves.

227

When given a garment, they may attempt to put it on backwards or upside down. Some just stand and appear blank as they have no concept of how to start the dressing process. This apraxia is most often noted with right occipitoparietal or bilateral occipitoparietal lesions. It is usually not noted in isolation and has elements of neglect and ideational apraxia.

Movement and task-specific praxis

Conceptual praxis is the associative knowledge of tool action while mechanical knowledge refers to the advantage tools offer. Frontal lobe degenerations cause conceptual praxis.

13: Agnosia

Agnosia is failure to recognize an object or sound with intact vision and hearing. Agnosia for taste and smell are rare. Agnosia for pain (SII cortical lesions) has recently been described.

Examining for agnosia

The patient is shown an array of common small objects and is asked to name them, describe their use and to pick out specific ones named by the examiner. If the patient is unable to do this visually, he or she is allowed to palpate the object and is asked the same questions. The patient is shown several different colors and asked to name them, match them with duplicates and then to arrange them in shades of increasing darkness or lightness. The patient is asked to walk to a specific location in a room when by doing so he or she would have to circumvent objects.

Visual agnosia

This is a disorder of higher cortical function in which an alert, intelligent, non-aphasic patient with normal visual perception cannot recognize a visual stimulus.

The patient is unable to name or describe the function of objects shown, but immediately identifies them by touch or noise (bell) or smell (rose). A patient with a nominal aphasia cannot name the object by any modality of presentation (visual object agnosia). The usual lesion for this deficit is the second and third gyri of the dominant occipital lobe and its adjacent white matter outflow tracts. The patient may also be unable to identify or match colors which is visual agnosia for colors.

There are several rather specific constellations of visual agnosia, which can be easily recognized and are quite striking.

Prosopagnosia

This is a visual agnosia in which the patient cannot recognize previously known faces and learn new ones but can do so through other modalities. The most striking example of this is a husband who cannot recognize his wife by sight, but does so immediately when she speaks. These patients are unable to recognize visual stimuli of a group that has subcomponents. Often, they can identify a class of a visual stimulus but are unable to identify a specific member within the generic class. The usual lesions associated with prosopagnosia are in the inferior or mesial visual association cortices of the lingual and fusiform gyri of the temporal lobe or their adjacent white matter. The problem lies in the patient's inability to access associated information from contextual memory banks.

Visual object agnosia

These patients are unable to recognize the generic class of an object. The finding is frequently clouded by both a nominal aphasia and alexia. Some patients complain that their vision is unclear when scanning the static object, but can recognize it when it is moved or rotated. This may be a defect of interpreting static low-contrast stimuli, which is overcome by movement which evokes high-contrast stimulus interpretations. The usual lesions identified are bilateral in the ventral and mesial part of the occipital second and third gyri.

Disorder of color perceptions

These are defects of color perception in all or part of the visual field with preservation of formed vision. Most often, the patient reports dull or washed out colors in the affected visual field, but when severe, he or she sees objects only as black or white. They have normal vision in the colorless portion of the visual field deficit. The usual lesion is in the left occipitotemporal cortex which may be associated with alexia. Rare patients with this deficit have lesions in the occipitotemporal white matter or superior occipital lobe.

Disorders of color naming

These patients can match colors, but are unable to name them. They have a concomitant right homonymous hemianopia, pure alexia, but intact color perception in the left visual field. The usual defect is between the occipital and temporal lobe of the dominant hemisphere. Some patients perform better when given the color's name and pointing them out rather than naming them on demand.

Visual agnosia for spaces

Patients with this deficit are incapable of maneuvering around obstructions or to go from one point to another. The usual lesions are bilateral in the posterior inferior parietal lobes (area 7). It may occur with unilateral lesions in which the patient will always turn to the ipsilateral side and will return to the starting point. This is usually a non-dominant parietal lesion. In its mildest form, migraine patients complain of visual disorientation when spreading depression affects the parietal lobe.

Tactile recognition

The patient must have normal sensation in both hands. He or she is then asked to close the eyes and several common objects are placed first in one hand and then the other. The patient is asked to describe their texture, size, shape and use. If he or she cannot accomplish this, the patient is allowed to look at, hear or smell the object. Complete absence of the ability to describe details of the object is usually astereognosis. If the patient can describe its size, shape and texture, but is unable to name it or describe its use by touch alone but does so with vision, the defect is tactile agnosia. It frequently coexists with visual object agnosia and is secondary to a lesion of the contralateral supramarginal gyrus. In a left-handed person, the defect could be in the corpus callosum (sensory information decoded in the right hemisphere cannot be transferred to the left supramarginal gyrus).

Auditory recognition

The patient has to have normal hearing. The examiner asks the patient to close the eyes and then uses a bell, rattles coins or whistles and the patient is asked to identify the sounds.

If a patient cannot recognize the sounds made by objects, but does so by sight or palpation he or she has auditory agnosia. These patients may have word deafness, so the instructions for the examination may have to be presented in written form. The usual lesion is in the posterior one-third of the dominant superior and medial temporal lobe.

The parietal lobe and disorders of the body scheme

Normally, a person knows at any given point in time the position of their body in space and its functional capacity. There is also a sense of the relation of the body in horizontal and vertical space. In the upright position, this sense of the midline of the body to a vertical axis is called the subjective visual vertical (SVV). The right parietal lobe is specialized for this body awareness, as it is for the patient's perception of near space (that which they can touch) and for space beyond their grasp. These abilities can be affected together or dissociated one from the other with lesions of the right parietal lobe.

Examination

The patient is asked to move the right and left hands. The examiner may then place his or her hands crossed behind the back and face the patient with the back turned and ask the patient to identify the right hand. The patient is asked to point out parts of his or her own body with each hand, with particular attention to fingers. The examiner may interlock the patient's fingers with his or her own and then ask the patient to identify individual digits. The examiner draws attention to the paralyzed or weak extremity. The examiner inquires if there is anything wrong with it and if it is part of the body. The patient is then asked to move it.

Many patients will have to think for a second or two to identify the right and left part of the body. If this is a problem, the examiner asks the patient to take his or her right hand and touch the left ear. Failing to cross the midline and to recognize the right from the left side of the body is usually a right parietal lesion.

Failure to identify a part of the body is autotopagnosia. Failure to recognize a side of the body is asomatotopagnosia. Failure to identify specific fingers is striking and is finger agnosia. The easiest finger to recognize is the thumb and the hardest is the fourth finger.

In non-dominant right parietal lobe lesions, the patient often neglects the left side of the body, is unaware of the deficit and may deny body parts. This often takes some bizarre turns as the patient may ascribe the hemiplegia to fatigue: "I used my arm yesterday and now it is resting." It may assume a negative quality: "Get this other arm out of my bed." Parts of an extremity may be denied. The patient agrees that the upper arm belongs to them, but the associated connected hand does not. As the stroke clears, patients recognize more of the affected body part. Anosognosia is denial of illness or dysfunction, which may also occur with deafness and blindness as well as motor function.

The opposite of denial of a body part is the phantom limb phenomenon of amputees. The patient imagines and feels the existence of the phantom. It is often exaggerated or distorted in size. It may appear on the stump of the extremity with the proximal component of the amputated part missing. It is frequently distorted, an example of which is one finger being elongated. Stroking the stump may evoke the phantom. The phantom is often painful and feels as if it is being twisted or crushed or stuffed into a shoe that is too small. There is clear physiologic reorganization of the sensory cortex in the absence of an extremity. Intact adjacent cortical areas innervate the prior territory of the amputated part. Phantoms shrink in size with time.

Sensory inattention

Inattention or perceptual rivalry refers to the lack of registration of a sensory stimulus when both homonymous parts of the body are stimulated simultaneously. The lesion is in the sensory pathways contralateral to the non-perceived stimulus. It occurs with visual, auditory and somatosensory stimulation.

Visual inattention

The examiner faces the patient with the arms held up. The patient is asked to fix the gaze between the examiner's eyes. The examiner than quickly flexes a forefinger and asks the patient which side moved. This is repeated in the contralateral visual field. The examiner then moves both fingers simultaneously. If there is visual inattention, the patient will not perceive the moving finger contralateral to the damaged occipital cortex. The examiner then moves the entire hand to see if this augmented visual stimulus can be appreciated. In dense lesions the deficit persists.

The patient is then asked to draw a flower, put the numbers in a clock or draw a house. The side that is neglected will be bare and frequently the objects and numbers will be crowded awkwardly into the good side. Neglect for spaces and constructional apraxia frequently coexist, which adds complexity to the interpretation of these observations.

The patient may not be able to see the hand in the deficient fields if it is stationary, but is able to do so when it moves (Riddoch's phenomenon). Conversely, if both hands are moving and the hand in the normal visual field stops, the patient may be able to see the hand in the abnormal field move when he or she could not formerly.

Auditory inattention

A patient must have approximately equal and normal hearing in both ears. He or she is then asked to close the eyes and indicate the side from which the noise is heard. The examiner clicks his or her fingers simultaneously and the patient will point to the side from which he or she hears the noise. The examiner can also utilize different loudness in each ear to sharpen the test. Keys can be shaken on the abnormal side and a click of the fingernail on the normal side. The patient will not perceive the louder noise.

Tactile inattention (Fig. 13.1)

The patient must have normal tactile sensation and be able to distinguish right from left. The patient is asked to close both eyes and then he or she is touched simultaneously on the dorsum of both hands. The patient will report only being touched on the side opposite the intact somatosensory system. If the patient is warned that both sides are going to be touched, he or she will be hyper alert and the sign missed. Further variants of the test are gently pricking both sides with a pin alternately. The examiner speeds up the alternate pricks and the patient will not perceive the side opposite the lesion. If the patient is asked to extend both hands and an object is placed into both, he or she will report only the side opposite the intact somatosensory system. The examiner watches how a patient manipulates an object placed into the palm of the hand. Normally, it is immediately dropped to the fingertips where it is palpated. A patient with peripheral or central sensory deficits will have a hard time getting the object to the fingertips. It will be awkwardly accomplished. This patient will have tactile inattention when given simultaneous stimulation. Tactile inattention is often frequently associated with dressing apraxia on the left side.

The parietal lobe and the motor cortex are intimately connected for use of the hand. High parietal lobe lesions frequently interfere with depth

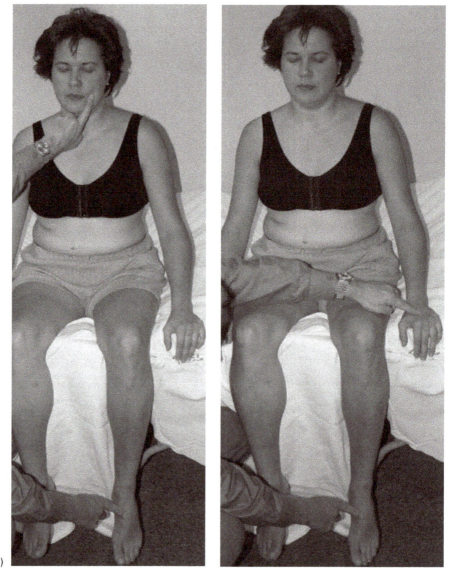

(a)

(b)

Fig. 13.1 Tactile inattention. (a) The examiner simultaneously lightly touches the face and the foot. The patient will not perceive the foot with right hemispheric lesions. (b) The examiner simultaneously lightly touches the hand and the foot. The patient will not perceive the hand with right hemispheric sensory lesions.

perception, precise hand use and occasionally cause Balint's syndrome, a component of which is "optic ataxia." The patient reaches for an object and consistently fails to grasp it because of misjudging its distance (undershooting it) although he or she sees it well. The patient has an inability to grasp an object with visual guidance. The inferior parietal lobe (area 7) directs gaze to new and important stimuli in the peripheral field and is also important for visually guided hand movements.

14: The Unconscious Patient

The content of consciousness is the patient's ability to remember, utilize and learn new information. It is the sum of all mental function. The level of consciousness is the degree of alertness or arousal. In general terms, the reticular activating system is the basis of arousal and the cerebral cortex for the content of consciousness. Full conscious activity requires at least one cerebral cortex and an intact brainstem.

The interplay between the reticular activating system and posterior thalamic and intralaminar nuclei determine the state of arousal. The ascending reticular activity system (RAS), which is important for consciousness, starts in the lateral medulla and receives afferents from all primary senses and the spinothalamic tract. The dorsal pons, periaqueductal gray and intralaminar nuclei of the thalamus are its most important subcortical components. The thalamic intralaminar nuclei have both cholinergic and GABAergic cells that regulate their activity. They project bilaterally to the cortex. Each cortical area is activated by a specific RAS projection. Disruption of the RAS at specific levels causes loss of consciousness or disorders of arousal.

As a general rule, patients with one functioning cerebral hemisphere are completely awake. Therefore, if the cortex is the area suspected of causing lethargy, the problem is usually metabolic, there has been a prior lesion of the other side or there is increased intracranial pressure. Most intracranial problems that alter consciousness do so by pressure on the periaquaductal gray of the midbrain (transtentorial herniation) or by destruction or pressure on the dorsal pons (basilar artery stroke). Thalamic lesions that affect the intralaminar nuclei cause loss of consciousness (acute hemorrhage). Thalamic lesions of the anteroventral (AV) and dorsomedial (DM) nuclei cause waxing and waning of consciousness. Rarely, patients are unconscious from bilateral medullary vascular lesions or trauma. Destructive hemispheric lesions have to be large enough to affect the contralateral hemisphere to cause decreased consciousness. Acute mass lesions cause more disorders of arousal than slowly evolving ones because the brain does not have time to accommodate the new increase of intracranial pressure. Small, strategically placed lesions of the dorsal pons or periaquaductal gray as well as bilateral brainstem lesions may cause profound coma.

Prior history in regard to the patient's coma is dramatically important. Unfortunately, a great number of patients who are examined have been found on the floor (FOF) with no helpful history. If resuscitated in the field by fire rescue, 95% of patients will never regain useful function. A good rule is if "found down" in the field "leave down."

The mode of onset of coma is extremely important. Sudden loss of consciousness is from medical causes from the heart or lung. If neurologic, it is a seizure, subarachnoid hemorrhage (SAH) or large embolus. The mechanism of loss of conscious from SAH is a cardiac arrhythmia from blood in the third ventricle rather than vasospasm. Rarely, an obstruction of the third ventricle from a colloid cyst or tumor can cause sudden loss of consciousness from positional change which causes internal hydrocephalus. This condition usually presents with severe positional headache. Coma over a few hours is usually secondary to a cerebral hemorrhage or swelling from a complete carotid occlusion. Neurologic patients usually vomit once from sudden increase of intracranial pressure that directly stimulates the vomit center of the area postrema which is located in the floor of the fourth ventricle. The initial increase of intracranial pressure is immediately buffered by overbreathing which causes vasoconstriction with a consequent decrease of cerebral blood flow (CBF). This is followed by collapse and shift of the ventricles, which displaces spinal fluid out of the brain and into the spinal subarachnoid space and a shift of the brain within the cranial vault. Several vomits suggest obstruction of a viscus of the gastrointestinal tract, while vomiting out of proportion to dizziness suggests brainstem ischemia. Coma of insidious onset suggests an expanding intracranial tumor. In general, sudden coma stems from cardiac arrhythmia or pulmonary embolus. Most neurologic coma is from increased intracranial pressure and transtentorial herniation.

Premonitory symptoms

No aura with loss of consciousness suggests a seizure, cardiac arrhythmia (Mobitz type II block), long QT interval or AV block. Rarely, an anterior communicating artery aneurysm ruptures into the third ventricle with consequent cardiac arrhythmia, loss of consciousness (Jefferson's syndrome) and often death.

Headache, vomiting, lethargy and focal neurologic signs all suggest an expanding intracranial lesion. If ataxia and diplopia are prominent, a cerebellar mass is most likely.

Systemic signs of weakness, anorexia and weight loss suggest metastasis or HIV with an opportunistic infection, while severe depression incriminates a drug overdose in a middle-aged person.

Cocaine causes two major neurologic syndromes: vasospasm and sudden increased pressure. A rupture of a pre-existing intracranial aneurysm or vascular malformation occurs in 20% of hemorrhages induced by cocaine. More commonly, vasospasm at 3 hours or later causes ischemic stroke or seizures. Phencyclidine (PCP) is suggested by self-destructive behavior and severe nystagmus. A patient with skin blisters found unconscious on the floor suggests phenobarbital overdose.

HIV is now stalking the world. Toxoplasmosis is the usual infection, but rarely causes coma and does not produce meningitis. In an HIV-positive patient who has meningitis, cryptococcus, tuberculosis, syphilis and deep fungal infection are the usual suspects, in that order. Computed tomography (CT) scan demonstrates basal ganglia involvement in cryptococcal infection which also causes stroke and basalar meningitis. Syphilis in the second stage is associated with meningitis and small strokes with ophthalmoplegia is characteristic of mucormycosis. A lung abscess should raise suspicion of aspergillosis and chronic leukemic conditions.

Alcoholism equals head trauma, subdural hematoma and, rarely, Wernicke–Korsakoff syndrome. In general, aphasia, sensory loss and visual field deficits are extremely rare with subdural hematomas. Fluctuating levels of consciousness occur as a result of expansion from rebleeding rather than from blood breakdown products and an increase of milliosmols in the subdural collection.

Trauma is particularly devastating in the elderly because of easy rupture of a dural bridging vein. Certainly, any coagulopathy, iatrogenic from coumadin or heparin, should always suggest intracranial hemorrhage as a cause of coma. Raccoon eyes and Battle's sign (discoloration of the mastoid) occur with basilar skull fracture. Subdural hematoma is a 6 hour to 2 day disease. Headaches, lethargy and spastic weakness are the predominant features. Epidurals have a triphasic course with loss of consciousness, a lucid interval and then decortication or decerebration occur. This is a 3 hour disease with blood in a convex rather than concave pattern on the CT scan.

Dehydration, obstetric cases (particularly unilateral seizures of the foot following delivery) Behçet's disease and hypercoagulable states all suggest sagittal sinus thrombosis. Bilateral thalamic hemorrhages on CT as well as direct evaluation of the sinuses by magnetic resonance venous (MRV) imaging establish this diagnosis.

The neurologic examination of the unconscious patient

Level of consciousness

Lethargy

A normal person answers questions quickly, holds attention to the matter at hand and remembers three out of three objects in 3 minutes. Calculation and general knowledge are as expected for the degree of education. The patient will perform well on visual praxis and follow the simple four-part command of "Take your right hand, touch your left ear, close your eyes and stick your tongue out." He or she will look quizzically at the examiner. When asked "Where did I touch you?" when the examiner touches his or her own face and the patient's hand (the face–hand test), the patient will answer "On the hand." The patient's affect will be appropriate for the situation.

Lethargy is a dangerous state. This is the earliest dangerous stage of any intracranial mass lesion and unfortunately patients are frequently discharged from the emergency room to collapse at home with this level of consciousness. The patient is slow to process information and appears sleepy. Stimulation arouses the patient to a state of complete alertness during which he or she processes information normally. Complex commands and calculations will be poorly accomplished and the patient has an excellent chance of failing the face–hand test. Patients again become lethargic if not stimulated. This state occurs with drug intoxications, metabolic failure and early midbrain pressure against the tentorium (almost always accompanied by focal neurologic signs). Our neurosurgical colleagues were the first to point out that patients with incipient transtentorial herniation may "walk and talk."

Obtundation

In this state, stimulation may raise the patient to a state of alertness in which he or she can follow commands poorly, but cannot carry out any complex function. The patient immediately reverts to his or her prior level of consciousness when the stimulation ceases. Bilateral cerebral hemispheric disease and compression of the upper brainstem as well as severe metabolic or drug intoxication cause obtundation. The pupillary light reflex is maintained and the eyes may be below the horizontal if the center for up gaze (r:MLF) in the midbrain is compressed.

Stupor

Vigorous stimulation usually only elicits a groan. There are no defensive maneuvers to avoid a painful stimulus. The eyes are below the horizontal (5–10°) if there is a structural lesion.

Coma

Patients are unconscious and do not respond to stimuli. They are immobile and incontinent. Pupillary, corneal and swallowing reflexes may be lost, but this is variable. The Glasgow coma scale quantifies degrees of eye opening, verbal and motor response in a patient with an altered level of consciousness.

Specific states of altered consciousness

Confusion and disorientation

The patient may be fully alert, but has no awareness of his or her condition and has deficits in orientation to time, place and person. Most people know the time within 15 minutes. Loss of place and person is most often seen in demented patients.

Delirium

These patients are unduly active, shout, gesticulate and speak incoherently. They hallucinate and are out of touch with their environment. Delirium occurs with toxic states and infection. It is common with alcohol withdrawal "delirium tremens" in which the patient often hallucinates that small green insects are attacking him or her. It is accompanied by severe autonomic dysregulation with tachycardia, hyperhidrosis and pupillary dilation.

Catatonia

The patient is psychotic, lies mute, immobile and unresponsive. He or she does not follow movements, is unaware of the surroundings and has a plastic rigidity of the extremities, which remain in the position in which they are placed by the examiner. Similar states have been described with frontal and hypothalamic lesions in association with other neurologic signs.

Akinetic mutism

The patient is motionless and speechless but appears awake. The patient may follow the examiner with the eyes. He or she has normal sleep–wake cycles and is always amnestic for the event. It occurs with lesions around the third ventricle or with involvement of the reticular formation in the upper brainstem.

Abulia

This occurs most often from subfrontal lesions seen with rupture and repair of an anterior communicating artery aneurysm. The patient initiates nothing and on vigorous stimulation may say "Yes" or "No." Curiously, a few patients have been described who initiate speech when given a toy telephone.

The locked-in syndrome

These patients have suffered complete destruction of the ventral pons. This lesion destroys the parapontine reticular formation (PPRF) so that horizontal gaze is lost. The centers for up gaze and blink are in the midbrain so that voluntary vertical gaze is possible. The patient is fully conscious. The usual lesion is a basilar artery or bilateral vertebral artery stroke.

Blood pressure

As a general rule, comatose patients with a low blood pressure have suffered a myocardial infarction, large pulmonary embolus or poisoning. Neurologic patients who are comatose have a high blood pressure from compression or ischemia of the lateral portion of the pontine tegmentum (the vasomotor center). The vasomotor center projects to the posterior hypothalamus, the nucleus magnus raptus of the medulla as well as to the intermediolateral columns of the spinal cord and the abdominal superior and inferior mesenteric ganglia. The net result is generalized vasoconstriction with an increase of central blood volume and peripheral vascular resistance. The increase of blood pressure, usually 220–210/120–110 mmHg, causes a slow pulse because of activation of the carotid sinus and the cardiodepressor nerves carried by ninth cranial nerve to the SA and AV nodes. The pulse is slow, usually 50–60 beats per minute, but full as a result of the sympathetic chronotropic effect on the heart. This is the basic physiology of the Kocher–Cushing reflex first described in a setting of increased intracranial pressure. As a patient herniates, either the midbrain (transtentorial) or rarely tonsillar level, the pulse becomes rapid and thready and the blood pressure falls to 90/60 mmHg.

Pulse rate

Atrial fibrillation and tachybrady arrhythmias are major causes of cerebral emboli. Most often, emboli cause transient ischemic episodes with focal deficits. Rarely, large red emboli (from the heart) will occlude enough blood vessels bilaterally in the cerebral cortex or the brainstem to cause loss of consciousness. A weak thready pulse is often seen in hemorrhagic shock, circulatory collapse and vasovagal syncope. Vagovagal syncope has a slow full pulse (the syncope by definition only lasts a few seconds). A weak irregular pulse is seen during cerebral herniation. Seizure disorders are often accompanied by tachycardia (anterior insular cortex focus).

Temperature

An accurate temperature is rarely obtained in an unconscious patient because of lack of oral access. Cold coma is most often seen in exposure to a cold environment. In general, hypoglycemia, renal and hepatic failure lower the temperature by 1°F. Severe hypothyroidism may lower the temperature to 92–93°F as does severe panhypopituitarism. Phenothiazines were originally developed to help in the movement of wounded soldiers (French, Vietnam war) and may lower the temperature to 92–93°F. Vascular accidents (meningohypophyseal trunk occlusion of the intracavernous carotid artery) or posterior hypothalamic tumors or hamartomas may also give severe hypothermia. The usual cause of hyperthermic coma is heat stroke. This usually requires a prior few days of hot humid weather in patients in non-air-conditioned houses. The temperature attained may be dramatic (109–112°F). Patients may feel cold as there is loss of shivering and sweating in concert with intense peripheral vasoconstriction. The cause of death is renal, cardiac and cerebral failure in a setting of disseminated intravascular coagulation (DIC). A temperature up to 104°F is most often infection. Above 105°F suggests anterior hypothalamic stroke, phenothiazine-based antidepressant overdoses, *Amanita* mushroom poisoning, isonicotinic hydrazide (INH) overdose and rarely blood in the ventricular system. Rarely, thyroid storm will raise the temperature above 105°F (generally accompanied by atrial fibrillation).

Respiratory patterns

Breathing patterns tell the examiner the level in the neuraxis at which the patient is functioning. A cortical breathing pattern of posthyperventilation apnea (PHVA) requires the cooperation of an awake patient to over-breathe. The patient takes three deep breaths and exhales quickly and forcibly (need to lower the Pco_2 by 18 mm/Hg). The fourth breath will be delayed (occurs at more than 20 seconds).

Cheyne–Stokes respiration

The patient has steady sustained hyperventilation with clear inspiratory and expiratory phases with superimposable apneic periods. Cheyne–Stokes respiration is frequently seen with congestive heart failure, uremia and hypertension. It is a mismatch or a delay in Pco_2 and Po_2 sensing by the cortex. Neurologic coma with Cheyne–Stokes respiration is most commonly seen at the level of the thalamus and basal ganglia from a hemorrhage. Much more commonly encountered is periodic breathing. In this pattern, there is a clear inspiratory and expiratory phase, but the apneustic spells are irregular. This also localizes to the thalamus and basal ganglia. Cheyne–Stokes returns as a terminal event from pressure on medullary respiratory neurons.

Central neurogenic hyperventilation

The normal breathing pattern is generally at 12–14 breaths per minute. Most nurses chart respiration at 20 breaths per minute which is central neurogenic hyperventilation (CNH). This is a pattern of steady hyperventilation, usually 20–40 breaths per minute. The examiner must be sure that there is no primary pulmonary disease that impedes oxygenation. The Po_2 has to be normal before this diagnosis can be made. If a structural lesion is involved, the pneumotatic center of the midbrain is disinhibited and its output drives pontine and medullary inspiratory neurons. Cerebral herniation, basilar artery stroke and cerebellar hemorrhages are the primary neurologic causes. Metabolic causes of CNH are diabetic ketoacidosis, lactic acidosis, uremia and poisoning. In diabetic ketoacidosis the inspiratory phase may be deeper (Kussmaul's breathing) than that noted from central causes.

Apneustic breathing

This pattern is one of deep inspiratory gasps and usually signifies pontine and medullary center dysfunction with approaching death. It is most often seen as the agonal breathing pattern of an unsuccessful cardiac resuscitation.

Medullary breathing patterns (ataxic, cluster and Biot's)

Ataxic breathing resembles that of Cheyne–Stokes, but the depth and regularity of inspiration is chaotic. Closely related is cluster breathing in which the patient may take several deep breaths with long apneic periods. Biot's breathing is couplet breathing, two breaths and then an apneic period.

Shallow rapid breathing is characteristic of patients in shock, who have suffered severe blood loss or are severely hypoglycemic and also occurs prior to the terminal event with central herniation.

General physical examination of the unconscious patient (Fig. 14.1)

A stiff neck suggests blood, pus or chemical irritation of the meninges. The patient's neck should be completely supple and on flexion the chin should

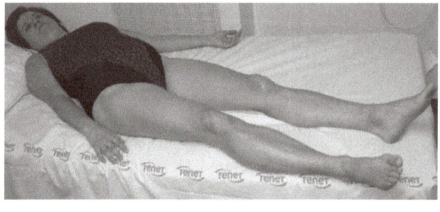
(a)

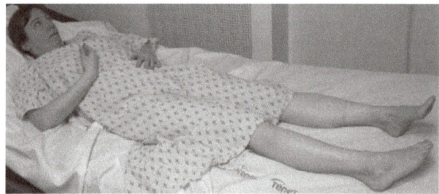
(b)

Fig. 14.1 Postures in comatose patients. (a) Parietal lobe. Note that the patient lies across the bed such that there is neglect of the left side of space. (b) Decorticate posture. Note the eyes are conjugately deviated to the side of the lesion. The right wrist fingers and arm are flexed and the right foot is slightly dropped and inverted. A left hemispheric lesion.

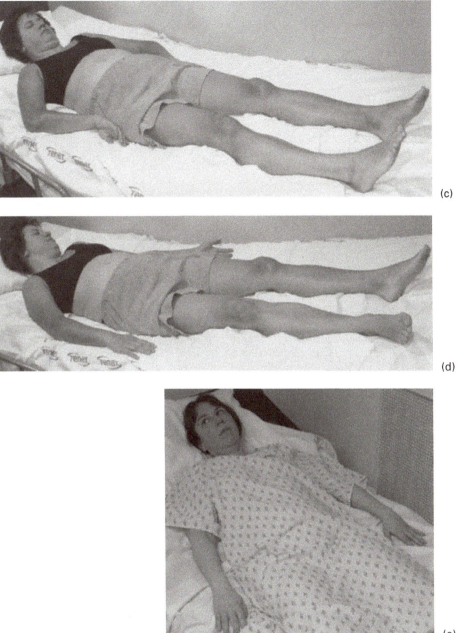

(c)

(d)

(e)

Fig. 14.1 (*cont'd*) (c) Decerebrate posture. The arms are adducted and internally rotated. The feet are in extension. (d) Corticospinal posture. The head and eyes are deviated to the left hemispheric lesion. The right arm is pronated with an adducted thumb. The left arm is supinated with an adducted thumb. The right leg is externally rotated. (e) Brainstem hemiparetic posture. The head and eyes are deviated to the right, the same side as the hemiparesis as noted from the adducted thumb. (*Cont'd on page 244*).

touch the chest wall. The examiner must be careful not to flex the neck until it has been cleared by X-ray in any suspected trauma (concomitant fractured spine). Brudzinski's sign is noted, which is a slight inward rotation of the foot and toes in an adult when the neck is flexed. A child may

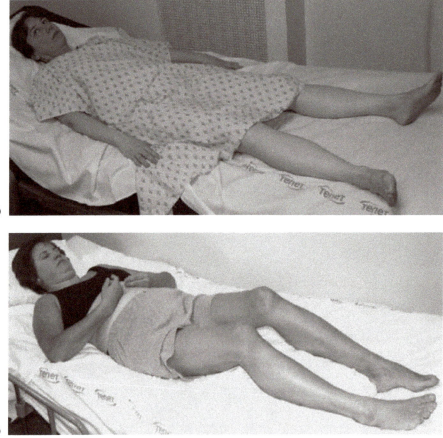

(f)

(g)

Fig. 14.1 (*cont'd*) (f) Bilateral corticospinal stroke. The eyes are deviated to the right and the right arm is pronated with an adducted thumb. The lesion is at the level of the left parapontine reticular formation. The left arm is pronated and the left foot externally rotated as a result of the brainstem corticospinal involvement. If the patient were "locked in", the eyes would be midline. (g) Bifrontal posture. Usually of long-standing. Flexed arms and legs. Apraxia of swallowing may be seen.

demonstrate classic flexion withdrawal of the lower extremities. Kerning's sign, inability to extend the leg after it is flexed onto the thigh, also demonstrates meningeal irritation. A stiff neck occurs with herniation of the cerebellar tonsils into the foramen magnum. There is usually torticollis when this occurs, the head and chin deviated to the contralateral side.

The entire neuraxis moves with neck flexion such that any pre-existing pressure on the third nerve will increase when this occurs. In a normal person, neck flexion cause dilation of the pupils which constrict to their normal size within a second or two (ciliospinal reflex). If there is pressure on the third nerve (uncal herniation), neck flexion will increase it further and the affected pupil will stay dilated (Forbes–Norris sign). This maneuver should only be performed once.

In an elderly or very ill patient, SAH may not cause neck stiffness for 24 hours. One must be careful not to confuse cervical spondylosis with neck stiffness from meningeal irritation.

Examination of the head and neck

Dysmorphisms of the head and neck are extremely helpful in diagnosis. A large head with frontal bossing suggests aqueductal stenosis. A shallow posterior fossa with low hair line suggests a Chiari malformation or craniovertebral junction defect. A large posterior fossa suggests the Dandy–Walker syndrome (congenital abnormality of the foramen of Lushka and Magendie associated with vermian atrophy). Wide-set eyes (hypertelorism) is frequently associated with absence of the corpus callosum, mental retardation and seizures.

Injuries are frequently hidden by hair. The examiner palpates for a fracture line, depression or "soggy" area that suggests contusion. A forehead contusion may be associated with a central cord injury which presents with arm greater than leg weakness. Battle's sign (ecchymosis of the mastoid bone) and the "raccoon eye" sign suggest basilar skull fracture. Burr holes should be sought as subdural hematomas may frequently reoccur in areas of prior drainage.

Middle ear infection is associated with intracranial abscess (usually in the cerebellum in children). Fluid behind the eardrum suggests basilar skull fracture.

During an epileptic attack the side of the tongue opposite the seizure focus may be bitten more severely than the contralateral side. It is rare for a true seizure patient to bite the tip of the tongue (most often seen with pseudoseizures).

In modern America, needle marks in veins suggest obvious intravenous drug abuse, its concomitant being HIV with attendant infection (notably toxoplasmosis, cryptococcus, tuberculosis, deep fungal infection and syphilis). Pulmonary edema and transverse myelitis in a lethargic patient is good evidence for recent intravenous heroin use.

Purpura or petechia in the skin suggest a coagulopathy. Petechiae over the chest wall suggest fat embolus, below the knee suggests Waldenström's macroglobulinemia (increase of blood viscosity and platelet malfunction), while hemorrhagic bullae are seen in patients who have been lying on the floor in a phenobarbital coma.

Broken bones, particularly long bones in young adults and adolescents, along with anterior chest wall petechia and a low Po_2 favor fat emboli. Surprisingly, older patients with fractures may have fat emboli because of an inability to transport fat (precipitation from chylomicrons) that obstructs small blood vessels and causes coma. This may also occur following hip replacement.

Posture in bed

Parietal lobe posture (see Fig. 14.1a)

The patient denies the left side of space. He or she will be found on the right side of bed at an angle (the feet more toward the midline). If the lesion is in the thalamus there is profound loss of position sense and the patient will be lying on the arm in a very awkward position.

Bifrontal lesions may cause a fetal posture with both arms and legs flexed. Decorticate posture is noted from lesion of the cortex and basal ganglion. The patient has flexed arms, extended legs and internally rotated feet. This will be associated with 2–3 mm pupils that react to light and periodic reaction.

Decerebrate posture occurs most commonly from structural brainstem damage. However, hypoglycemia, hepatic failure, hypoxia and phenobarbital intoxication cause reversible decerebration. The usual lesions are pressure on or destruction of the midbrain between the superior colliculus and the pons. The patient has extended, adducted and internally rotated arms with extension of the feet. The ankles cannot be dorsiflexed. A common mistake is to overlook the significances of even a small degree of adduction and internal rotation of an upper extremity which represents decerebrate rigidity.

Both decorticate and decerebrate postures are elicited by painful compression of the supraorbital nerve or sternum.

External rotation of the leg and pronation of the arm

This leg posture signifies pyramidal tract damage of the contralateral side (unless, of course, the hip is broken or dislocated in which case the leg is shorter). The head is often deviated to the side of the lesion if the frontal eye fields are involved. If the eyes are deviated to the side of the hemiparesis, the lesion is in the pons.

Opisthotonus in an adult is most often seen in tetanus that occurs with intravenous drug abuse. If severe, only the occiput and the heels will touch the bed.

A flexion posture away from the light suggests meningeal imitation. Compression of the patient's closed eyes is painful with meningeal irritation. Inability to compress the eye (carried out carefully and slightly) suggests an increase of intracranial pressure. This is most common with SAH.

The doll's head maneuver and ice-water caloric test

A comatose patient has lost cortical fixation reflexes, which allows the examiner to examine oculovestibular reflexes. The purpose of these ocular reflexes are to foveate (hold gaze on an object) while the head is moving. In a comatose patient with an intact brainstem (non-structural lesion between the medullary vestibular nuclei and the third nerve nuclei of the midbrain), turning the head to the right will cause the eyes to conjugately deviate to the left and the opposite will occur on turning the head to the left. Also, if the head is extended, the eyes deviate conjugately downward while in flexion the reverse occurs.

A stronger stimulus for the same maneuver is the use of ice-water calorics. The head is flexed 30° and 1 mL ice water is gently irrigated into the external auditory canal. The eyes will slowly deviate to the side of the irrigation and will then return to the midline within 2 minutes. The reverse will occur when the opposite ear is irrigated. The head must be extended 60° below the horizontal and both external canals irrigated simultaneously with warm water to evaluate vertical gaze. If ice-water calorics are intact, this means that there is no structural lesion from the medulla (vestibular nuclei) to the midbrain (third nerve). Deep coma from severe metabolic depression will also freeze the eyes. An intact reflex requires stimulation of the eighth nerve vestibular complex, which utilizes the medial longitudinal fasciculus (MLF) to coordinate excitation of the ipsilateral sixth nerve of the lower pons and the contralateral third nerve of the midbrain. There is reciprocal inhibition of the contralateral sixth nerve and ipsilateral third nerve. If the medial longitudinal fasciculus is interrupted, the eyes do not deviate conjugately. The side of the stimulated ear will deviate ipsilaterally, but the contralateral eye will not cross the midline.

The area under the superior colliculus in the midbrain, the rostral interstitial nucleus of the MLF (riMLF) coordinates vertical gaze. Pressure on this midline ocular area or its destruction will paralyze up gaze. This is a most helpful sign because it means a structural cause of coma. The downward deviation is often subtle, but must be sought assiduously.

Ocular position and ocular movement

This part of the examination is most helpful. The level of the lesion and often its cause can be instantly diagnosed if eye movements and position are examined properly. Eyes that are below the horizontal suggest a structural lesion that affects up gaze. Deviation of the eyes to one side with contralateral hemiplegia is a lesion of the frontal eye fields and its adjacent motor territory. Look at the position of the eyes on the accompanying CT or magnetic resonance imaging (MRI) scan. Cortical eye deviation lasts only for 24 hours and often less. If the eyes are deviated to the side of the hemiparesis, the lesion is in the pons. Cortical eye deviation can be vestibular ocular reflex across the midline or driven over with ice-water calorics. Pontine deviation cannot be altered by any maneuver. A skew deviation means that the eyes are not on the same vertical plan. If the lesion is in the brainstem (medullary or pontine), it is on the side of the down eye. If the lesion is at a basal ganglion or thalamic level, it will be contralateral to the down eye. Skew deviations are most common with cerebellar or pontine lesions.

Severe esotropia (both eyes adducted) suggests acute sixth nerve palsy from increased intracranial pressure. The nerves are trapped under the petroclinoid ligament (Dorello's canal). The eyes will also be slightly below the horizontal.

Eyes that are severely adducted and are looking down at the tip of the nose are associated with a thalamic lesion. This may occur with only one eye.

247

Ocular bobbing tells the examiner that the lesion is in the pons. The eyes are conjugately driven down and then float up. Ocular dipping has the same localizing value but the physical finding is just a quick downward conjugate movement of the eye with a rapid return to the normal position. These pontine eye signs are associated with pinpoint pupils (less than 0.5 mm), central neurogenic hyperventilation and complete or partial decerebration. Nystagmus retractorius is rare (all eye muscles contract simultaneously), which the examiner notes by the rhythmic variation of the palpebral fissures. This finding is associated with lesions of or around the periaqueductal gray of the midbrain. Eyes that are driven down and to one side suggest tonsillar herniation to the side of the down eyes.

Upbeat nystagmus localizes a lesion to the pontomedullary junction or the superior vermis. These patients may demonstrate decerebrate posture of the arms with flexed posture of the legs. Downbeat nystagmus signifies a lesion of the posterior fossa. Roving eye movements are characteristic of bicortical damage. Metronomic movements, the eyes pause at the limit of their excursion, are secondary to cerebellar Purkinje cell dysfunction, usually from an anoxic event such as a cardiac event.

The pupils

As a general rule, in most patients with toxic or metabolic causes of coma, the pupillary light reflexes are spared. This is an important differential point between metabolic and structural causes of coma.

Widely dilated pupils (7–9 mm) that do not react to light occur in midbrain lesions. They may also be seen in cortical stimulation from cocaine or amphetamine. Midbrain lesions or those that affect the third nerve or its complex do not react to light. A smaller pupil (4–7 mm) that does not react to light may also be caused by a midbrain lesion. Cadaveric midbrain pupils are 3 mm and do not respond to any form of stimulation. Cat's eye pupils (elliptical) have been described in midbrain head trauma. A dilated oval pupil is most often seen with compression of the third nerve. Each part of the Edinger–Westphal (EW) nucleus has responsibility for a component of the iris. Partial lesions of the EW nucleus cause damage and therefore weakness of a component of the iris. This changes the radial contraction of the pupil and it becomes oval. An oval pupil has been reported with partial third nerve palsy, diabetes and syphilis.

Unilateral pupillary dilation in a patient who has sustained head trauma, deep cerebral hemorrhage or a middle cerebral artery (MCA) stroke with edema in association with lethargy is a sign of transtentorial herniation. The dilation is on the side of the lesion. The hemiparesis is on the contralateral side as the opposite cerebral peduncle is compressed against the tentorium which causes ipsilateral weakness (Kernohan's notch syndrome). If both pupils are dilated, herniation is often complete and there is bilateral third nerve compression or a secondary Duret's hemorrhage of the midbrain.

Normal pupils react briskly to light. Pressure on the third nerve or a nuclear third nerve palsy slows the speed of pupillary contraction. The examiner watches the speed of constriction when the eyelids are lifted as well as when they are stimulated with a bright light. A nuclear third nerve palsy occurs from infarction of the interpeduncular artery from the top of the basilar artery or pressure on the midbrain. A nuclear third nerve is associated with:

1 bilateral ptosis;
2 bilateral pupillary dilation;
3 failure of up gaze because of damage to the afferent supply to the superior rectus muscle;
4 is not so rare as once believed.

A good rule is that drug overdose paralyzes the extraocular muscles before the pupils. Upward herniation (lesions in the posterior fossa) paralyzes up gaze prior to the pupils. In this situation, the superior vermis is pushed upwards and forward which compresses the collicular plate. This also was thought to be rare until the advent of MRI.

Pupils that are 2–3 mm but react briskly to light suggest a lesion at the level of the thalamus or basal ganglia. Pinpoint pupils less than 0.5 mm are characteristic of pontine lesions. This scenario is often accompanied by decerebrate rigidity and CNH. The examiner must be aware that pilocarpine, parathion and narcotics cause similar pupillary construction, but usually not to the same degree. Meperidine only affects the pupil two-thirds of the time. Lateral medullary and posterior hypothalamic lesions cause 1 mm pupils.

The cranial nerves

The fundi

This part of the examination is extremely important in the unconscious patient. Papilledema does not occur in infants under 1 year of age nor in most elderly patients after 65 years of age. Sutures split in the former and the ravages of life with consequent atrophy occur in the latter. Papilledema takes 2–3 days to develop unless there has been severe head trauma with loss of cerebral autoregulation that causes increased blood flow to the eye and brain. This again is most often seen in young patients who have suffered severe head trauma.

Blood between the macula and the disk may be seen with SAH (Torsten's syndrome). It is caused by a sudden increase in intracranial pressure and rupture of preretinal veins. The blood may move with head position. In the past it was thought to occur from leakage of blood through subarachnoid pathways and under the dura of the optic nerve. Approximately 20% of aneurysms are bilateral. The side in which the hemorrhage is seen is the side of the aneurysm that bled.

249

CHAPTER 14
The Unconscious Patient

Visual fields cannot be tested in a comatose patient. In stuporous patients, the patient will not blink on the side of a visual stimulus. Facial weakness in a comatose patient is noted by flattening of the nasolabial fold, less wrinkling of the forehead and a weak lower eyelid. The buccinator muscle is weak and the cheek opposite the side of the lesion will be weak. Expiration will blow out the cheek on the weak side and inspiration will suck it in. Pressure over the supraorbital nerve (in the notch of the eyebrow) is painful and the weak side of the face does not grimace when this is stimulated.

The corneal reflex is absent in coma. It is a segmental reflex, and if absent on the stimulated side suggests a midpontine pathology. It is frequently lost in patients with complete hemianalgesia from deep-seated basal ganglia hemorrhage or upper brainstem lesions. A cornea mandibular reflex, in which the jaw deviates to the contralateral side with ipsilateral corneal stimulation, signifies severe cortical degeneration. Loss of facial sensation ipsilaterally with loss of sensation below the clavicle contralaterally is characteristic of lower brainstem lesions, particularly Wallenberg's syndrome from thrombosis of the vertebral or posterior inferior cerebellar artery.

Movement of the extremities

Patients with structural lesions anywhere in the course of descending motor pathways demonstrate much less movement on the side opposite the lesion than the normal side. In general, the deeper the brain lesion the more cerebral brain shock occurs with a contralateral flaccid hemiparesis. The cerebral cortex is biased toward inhibition, therefore acute lesions may give hyperactive reflexes. A patient with cerebellar hematoma typically presents with quadriparesis rather than quadriplegia and if untreated rapidly progresses to coma.

If the patient is not moving, hard pressure applied over the supraorbital nerve will stimulate a grimace. Hard pressure over the center of the sternum will stimulate movements of the arms or legs. If the corticospinal tract is intact, noxious stimuli elicit movements away from the afferent input. Movements of individual fingers and toes are absolute evidence of an intact pyramidal system. Patients with corticospinal tract dysfunction when stimulated on flexor or extensor surfaces demonstrate flexion and adduction of the arms and shoulders. Noxious stimulation of the lower extremities causes extension and adduction of the lower limbs.

Tone is helpful in determining the site of an intracranial lesion. Both arms are raised together and then released. Normally, the fall is checked and slowed, but the arm falls unchecked if it is weak. The legs are flexed at the knee by the examiner. They are then released. A normal leg will maintain the flexed position with the sole on the bed while the paralyzed one will rapidly slide back to its initial position.

250

Involuntary movements in unconscious patients

Convulsions

Postictal paralysis (Todd's paralysis) frequently follows a focal seizure. The paralysis is almost always secondary to a structural lesion. It usually lasts from minutes to hours and rarely for days. Recently, seizures in speech areas have been reported to cause deficits in language function for several weeks. The mechanism is increased inhibition from intracortical GABAergic interneurons and inhibitory volleys from the cerebellum. It has been described from area 6 seizures (motor inhibitory strip of Hines). The paralysis is not caused by metabolic failure of the seizurogenic area. In general, seizures from metabolic causes are not focal. Focal seizures from hypoglycemia are an exception. Perfusion failure from cardiac arrhythmia produces a generalized seizure in more than 90% of patients. Focal brain disease equals focal seizures. Leg area seizures in pregnant women suggest sagittal sinus thrombosis or in an elderly patient a parasaggittal meningioma. Cocaine abuse often causes focal vasospasm and seizures. If there is a hemorrhage from cocaine abuse, 20% of patients harbor an underlying vascular malformation. Minor twitching of an extremity has localizing value. Repeated focal convulsions that recruit more muscles of the extremity with each seizure suggest venous cortical infarction.

Myoclonus

Myoclonus is a rapid asymmetric movement of an extremity or joint. It is generally divided into the following:
1   corticoreticular, in which a cortical motor spike precedes the movement;
2   brainstem (nucleus gigantocellularis);
3   segmental (origin is the spinal cord).
Most often, generalized myoclonus in an unconscious adult will be from anoxia, a hyperosmotic state, uremia or cyclosporine.

Decerebrate attacks

These are waves of decerebration that occur spontaneously or with stimulation such as tracheostomy care. Brainstem compression from transtentorial herniation, basilar artery stenosis or occlusion are major causes. Reversible decerebration may occur with hepatic coma, anoxia and phenobarbital intoxication. It may be unilateral and alternate with decortication. If this occurs, the lesion is on the side opposite the decerebration.

Rigors or tremors

Hard to describe tremulous movements occur with blood or pus in the ventricular system as well as with cyclosporine, uremia and other metabolic failures. Fasciculations across the chest wall are seen with pontine hemorrhage.

Coordination

This cannot be tested in a comatose patient. Ataxic movements during stimulation or localization of a painful stimulus can occasionally be seen in obtunded and stuporous patients.

Reflexes

This component of the examination is very helpful. Reflexes are frequently absent in comatose patients or are decreased on the side opposite a deep hemorrhage at basal ganglia or thalamic levels (brain shock). They may be increased in pure cortical lesions. Most metabolic coma patients have lost reflexes with the exception of hypocalcemia and hypomagnesemia. They are increased in the brainstem phase of hepatic insufficiency concomitantly with decerebrate rigidity and small pupils.

Selective necrosis of brainstem nuclei

This occurs most often in infants, children and adolescents although it has been reported in adults. These patients have no oculocephalic eye movements, or branchial muscle function which includes the gag reflex. There is no spontaneous movement and all extremities are stiff. Although some automatic movements with stimuli remain, there is autonomic disinhibition with wide fluctuations of blood pressure and cardiac rate, and there is loss of spontaneous respiration.

Bihemispheral coma

These patients are unresponsive to noise, bright light or voice. They respond to painful stimuli but localize it poorly although they regain spontaneous movement of the extremities. In general, the pupils are normal or small and react to light. Eye movements move from side to side and are midline. Some patients have upward deviated eyes. Patients have hyperactive doll's eye movements as a result of loss of ocular fixation reflexes. Vertical eye movements are present to vestibular ocular reflex maneuvers but may be difficult to deviate downwards if the eyes are fixed in upward gaze. The gag reflex is intact as are branchial innervated movements. Spontaneous blink and swallow reflexes are present.

Metabolic coma

In general, there are no focal neurologic deficits with the exception of hypoglycemia, hepatic failure, anoxia and phenobarbital poisoning. These latter may cause reversible decerebration and alternate decerebration and decortication. If the latter is the case, a structural lesion should always be sought on the side opposite the decerebration. Pupil size and reactivity vary widely in metabolic coma states and certainly are not as reliable a physical sign as a cranial nerve palsy. There are no sensory or visual field deficits while adventitial movements such as myoclonus and seizures are common. The reflexes are most often depressed with the exception of hypocalcemia and hypomagnesemia.

The examiner's major purpose in evaluation of a comatose patient is to determine its cause as quickly as possible as a great number of structural or metabolic entities are treatable. The examiner must immediately determine if loss of consciousness is a result of a metabolic or structural cause. If the former, its specific etiology must be sought and if the latter the level of involvement of the neuraxis and its pathology should be elucidated.

Unfortunately, the situation becomes complicated when a lesion causes a prolonged seizure with attendant acidosis, anoxia and dehydration or when anoxia and hypotension lead to widespread structural damage. The status of the patient's central nervous system prior to the new event may determine the level of consciousness.

The important point is that the examiner has a clear plan of evaluation. The vital signs above often give the differential diagnosis.

15: The Autonomic Nervous System

General inspection

The skin frequently reflects autonomic dysregulation. Livido reticularis (a blue lacy pattern), dusky cyanosis and poor capillary refill tell the examiner that capillary circulation of the extremity is not regulated properly. There is a delicate interplay between sympathetic vasoconstriction and the release of vasoactive neuropeptides in the skin. The tips of the fingers and toes are important for thermoregulation and have a high blood flow. The deep circulation to muscles, adventitial tissues and bone is the core of the nutritive blood supply. Dysfunction of the sympathetic nervous system at this level causes the atrophy and dystrophy of chronic regional pain syndrome (CRPS). The peripheral nerves carry sympathetic fibers to the extremities and all components of their tissue. Almost all peripheral neuropathies, particularly the small fiber axonal ones, are associated with cold extremities. Sympathetic tone increases and decreases minute by minute. Large dilated veins on an extremity that do not vary in diameter during the day suggest loss of this tone. A flushed warm extremity suggests loss of sympathetic tone. Inspiration blocks cutaneous thermoregulatory blood flow. Extremely red ears and facial flushing are manifestations of sympathetic paralysis and the release of vasoactive neuropeptides on the corresponding blood vessels (neurogenic edema). These neuropeptides paralyze smooth muscle and increase capillary leakage.

Complete sympathetic lesions result in absence of sweating while irritative lesions may increase sweating. There is no denervation hypersensitivity with resulting hyperhidrosis after sympathetic denervation. Excessive hyperhidrosis has a central nervous system origin and may be seen after a cortical or posterior hypothalamic stroke.

A peripheral Horner's syndrome is seen from loss of sympathetic innervation that derives from the C8–T1 dermatome and follows the internal carotid artery to the eye. The T2 sympathetic dermatome selectively innervates the arm.

Cardiovascular reflexes

Postural hypotension

The usual blood pressure response on standing is a drop of 5–10 mmHg systolic pressure with an increase of 5 mmHg diastolic pressure. This is effected through cardiodepressor nerves (ninth cranial nerve) that sense a decrease of pressure (carotid sinus) and then increase the heart rate to compensate for this pressure drop. Following this increase in heart rate there is a relative bradycardia. A patient who has a fall of more than 20–30 mmHg systolic pressure on standing has an abnormal response. If there is no corresponding increase in pulse rate, the parasympathetic arm of the autonomic system is also involved (there is also no variance of the R-R interval on electrocardiogram (ECG)).

Blood pressure response to pressure stimuli

Mental calculations, sustained handgrip or exposure to cold increase blood pressure. Less than 10 mmHg rise in systolic pressure is abnormal. Peripheral and central causes of sympathetic dysfunction affect these tests. The sympathetic nervous system is centrally regulated such that stimulation of one extremity is reflected by responses of the other extremities (effected through the posterior hypothalamus and the nucleus magnus raphus of the medulla).

Heart rate response

The change of posture from the supine to standing increases heart rate which is effected by the parasympathetic system. Thus, peripheral autonomic neuropathies often will affect both the sympathetic and parasympathetic response. These are principally diabetes, acute intermittent porphyria, paraneoplastic diseases, autoimmune small fiber neuropathies, amyloid and hereditary autonomic sensory motor neuropathy (HSAN I–IV).

Massage of the carotid sinus stimulates vagal receptors and initiates consequent parasympathetic activity. The right carotid is usually more sensitive and dangerous to stimulate as bradycardia and severe hypotension may occur in sensitive patients.

The heart rate varies with breathing; this is known as sinus arrhythmia.

The Valsalva maneuver

The patient exhales against a closed glottis, which causes the blood pressure to drop and the heart rate to increase (decreased cardiac return with compensatory heart rate increase). Opening the glottis increases cardiac return, which results in an overshoot of the resting blood pressure with a consequent slowing of heart rate. Afferent or efferent parasympathetic lesions block the response.

Skin responses

Erythema

The triple response of Lewis comprises a blanch, wheal and flare. The patient's skin is stroked with the back of a reflex hammer. There is first a blanch, which is the result of direct stimulation of the sympathetic nerve endings that surround cutaneous blood vessels (vasoconstriction). Then a wheal appears, slight edema from the mechanical stimulation of the skin that releases substance P (SP) and calcitonin gene-related peptide (CGRP) from C fibers that also innervate skin vessels. The former (SP) causes a 500-μm hole in the capillary endothelium with consequent extravasation of plasma, and the latter (CGRP) paralyzes smooth muscle. The flare is caused by an axon reflex. Depolarization of C fibers progresses to other C fiber terminals at branch points, which releases SP in concert with those mechanically stimulated. This released SP interacts with the mast cells that surround skin blood vessels and cause them to release histamine which dilates the skin capillaries. The response is lost in any neuropathic condition that damages C fibers in the skin, which in general are Guillain–Barré syndrome (GBS) and other autoimmune neuropathies. The response is exaggerated in complex regional pain syndrome. The response may also be increased below a spinal lesion, which thus demarcates its level.

Temperature

In acutely sympathetically denervated areas, the skin or extremity is warm because of loss of sympathetic vasoconstrictor tone. This is helpful in brachial and lumbar plexus lesions where the sympathetics may be involved and in patients with CRPS. In chronic sympathetic denervation, the extremity is frequently cold because there has been up-regulation of α-adrenoreceptors on the denervated blood vessels which constrict to circulating norepinephrine from the adrenal glands.

Pilomotor response

Each hair is erect when its follicular base contracts. Piloerection is produced by a mechanical stimulus or cold metal on a warm body part. This response is very active in states of heightened sympathetic activity such as opioid withdrawal ("cold turkey") and in CRPS.

Scrotal responses

Touching the scrotum with cold metal causes vermicular contraction of the dartos scroti muscle which does not elevate the testicles. The cremasteric reflex (elicited by stroking the inner thigh) elevates the testicles. The scrotal response is absent in sympathetic denervation.

The sweating test

Laser Doppler fluxmetry and sophisticated thermography have supplanted this test. As a general rule, hyperhidrosis is an overactive central sympathetic innervation. A cold clammy extremity occurs in chronic peripheral denervation where Canon's law applies, while a flushed, warm, dry extremity is indicative of sympathetic denervation.

Thoracic tumors, primarily cancer of the lung, may be announced by segmental hyperhidrosis as the cancer grows into or irritates the segmental sympathetic supply.

Examination of bladder function

Voluntary initiation of micturition is generated from the second frontal convolution and is suppressed by the paracentral lobule of the parietal lobe so that micturition occurs at the proper time. Lesions of the superior frontal lobe and anterior cingulate gyri may cause unawareness of bladder fullness and incontinence. Bilateral cortical dysfunction from degenerative disease, strokes, tumor or hydrocephalus can cause cortical precipitate micturition. Vesical sensation can be felt at 100–150 mL at a pressure of 6 cm H_2O. Bladder fibers pass to the pontine micturition center which then project to the cervical micturition center at C8–T1 (the ciliary center of Budge). The detrusor muscle of the bladder wall must discharge with an open external sphincter to effect micturition. The pontine and cervical micturition centers coordinate this function. Posterior lesions of the frontal lobes may cause spasticity of the striated muscles of the external sphincter with consequent bladder retention. Incomplete lesions of the upper motor neuron pathways to the detrusor muscle cause a neurogenic bladder that is small and is associated with frequency and urgency. In a neurogenic bladder, the trigone (its sensory component) reflexly fires because of the increased pressure from this thick-walled small bladder. A complete spinal cord transaction causes paralysis of the bladder with overflow incontinence. This changes to a reflex bladder (neurogenic) over 6 weeks to 2 months which then automatically empties but may be induced to contract by abdominal pressure. Lesions of the sacral cord (S1–S5) or the cauda equina cause a flaccid large bladder (400–600 mL) with "overflow incontinence." Associated with loss of the parasympathomimetic supply of S1–S4 to the detrusor muscle, there is concomitant somatic sensory loss in the S2–S4 dermatomes. Tabes dorsalis destroys both the sympathetic and parasympathetic components of the bladder innervation which causes painless bladder enlargement with overflow incontinence (the bladder usually contains 400–600 mL urine).

The history of bladder function is often poorly taken. A normal patient should not get up more than once per night and at most twice. Inability to initiate micturition, a divided urinary stream, dribble and poor force all suggest prostatic obstruction. An insensible bladder suggests a severe peripheral neuropathy, cytomegalovirus (CMV) infection in an HIV patient, or tabes dorsalis. Inability to interrupt voiding by voluntary sphincter control suggests a lesion of Onuf's nucleus (S2–S4) of the conus medullaris (not involved in amyotrophic lateral sclerosis (ALS), but involved in multiple system atrophy). Urgency and frequency with the inability to initiate micturition is dyssynergia between the detrusor muscle (Onuf's nucleus S2–S4 and the external sphincter of the penis innervated by L5–S1). This is most often seen with thoracic and cervical cord demyelinating lesions. A good clinical test of detrusor function is to have the patient take a deep breath while urinating. If the detrusor is not functioning, the stream will stop as abdominal pressure has been relieved.

A complete lower motor neuron bladder is large, devoid of feeling, does not contract reflexly and is hypercompliant. Voiding requires straining and is not complete. The usual pathologies for this condition are autonomic peripheral neuropathy, cauda equina or conus medullaris lesions.

An upper motor neuron bladder is small, insensible, hyperreflexic (contracts with a smaller than normal urine volume), is hypocompliant (does not expand enough for the intravesicular pressure) and has a hyperactive sphincter. The patient has reflex voiding.

When studied carefully most bladder lesions are mixed. The associated neurologic signs and symptoms give the examiner the correct answer. Absent reflexes, a peripheral neuropathy, primarily to pinprick and cold, suggest a small fiber neuropathy. Proprioceptive and vibration loss, areflexia and an Argyll Robertson pupil is characteristic of tabes dorsalis. It may be from diabetes rather than syphilis and is then known as pseudotabes. In general, cauda equina, conus medullaris and peripheral neuropathies cause a decrease or loss of bladder sensation. This results in a high intravesicular pressure and a normal to slightly increased capacity. It is an insensible atonic bladder that has low pressure (distends easily to an increase of pressure), has no spontaneous contractions and contains a high residual urine.

Cerebral lesions often cause precipitate micturition. This is particularly evident in normal pressure hydrocephalus (NPH). Degenerative disease usually causes reflex micturition at low bladder capacity although there may be bladder retention. Bladder sensation is normal, there is a reduced capacity and precipitate micturition is the rule. An overflow incontinence does not occur in patients with high spinal or cerebral lesions. A patient with a high cervical cord lesion may have precipitate micturition during a Valsalva maneuver.

The rectum

Acute lesions of the conus medullas or the cauda equina (pelvic nerves) cause fecal incontinence. There will be laxity of both the internal and external sphincter and the anal reflex will be absent. Acute spinal cord injuries cause spinal shock with incontinence of the anal sphincters. High spinal or pontine lesions may cause spasticity of anal sphincters. Major motor seizures may cause fecal incontinence although urinary incontinence is more common.

Sexual function

Prior to a neurologic work-up, patients with sexual dysfunction need to be screened for depression, hypothyroidism and a pituitary prolactinoma that causes a low testosterone and a high prolactin level. Autonomic failure from neuropathy or that which occurs with central autonomic failure such as Shy–Drager, striatonigral degeneration or multiple system atrophy destroys sexual function. Spinal cord tumors slowly expanding in the conus medullaris may cause dissociated sexual function. A patient may be able to achieve an erection, but is unable to ejaculate or the reverse. Demyelinating disease and a syrinx may cause similar symptoms. Rarely, root disease causes sexual disfunction. Potency may be affected prior to bladder function in males with spinal cord disease.

Psychically induced erections are mediated by the parasympathetic hypogastric nerves. The sacral roots control reflex erection. Spinal lesions as well as lymphoma, polycythemia and the new 5′ esterase inhibitors may cause prolonged painful erections (priapism). Spinal lesions above T12 may cause impotence with intact reflex erection, but without ejaculation. Impotence with retained reflex erection and ejaculation is often psychiatric. The bulbocavernosus reflex evaluates the sacral cord and is performed by pinching the glans penis which causes contraction of the bulbocavernosus muscle behind the scrotum. Cauda equina lesions abolish erection, ejaculation and sexual sensation as well as impair sensation in the perineum.

Conclusions

Neurology has changed drastically over the last 25 years. It is now a specialty that not only diagnoses illnesses but treats them. There is a general notion that a neurologist "diagnoses everything, but treats nothing." This is completely incorrect. A neurologist does diagnose everything and now treats everything. Clot busting with urokinase and tPA are routine. Stenting and angioplasty of arteries in both the anterior and posterior circulations are commonly performed. Surgery for refractory seizure disorders is the new frontier for epilepsy. The return of surgery for Parkinson's disease and other severe movement disorders is extending the useful life of these patients when existing therapies fail. Gene therapy for enzyme defects and storage disorders is underway. The use of transcortical brain stimulation to activate and inactivate functional loops of the brain will change concepts of brain function and unleash opportunities for rehabilitation. The use of immune suppressants and immunomodulators as well as plasmapheresis and intravenous immunoglobulin is changing the management of the immune disorders that affect the peripheral and central nervous systems. The use of neurotrophic factors to save cells that may be struggling for survival is starting. Great advances have been made in understanding mechanisms that underlie chronic pain states. This may lead to therapies to restore normal dorsal horn and central pain projecting neurologic function and thus relieve intractable pain conditions.

Magnetic encephalography (MEG) allows an online time analysis of a specific neurologic process. Functional magnetic resonance imaging (MRI) demonstrates which loops of a circuit are involved in a specific function. Positron emission tomography (PET) scanning demonstrates components of active functional loops, which transmitters are being utilized, as well as the affinity and distribution of specific receptors for specific functions.

The widespread use of computed tomography (CT) and MRI by primary care physicians, neurosurgeons and psychiatrists seems to lessen the need for a good neurologic history and detailed examination but MRI does not visualize bone well and CT does not image soft tissue well. At least 50% of patients have obvious sciatic severe involvement that cannot be visualized. There are some tricky features of migraine headache that can be visualized, but most cannot. The history enables this diagnosis. A great deal of the phenomenology seen in neurologic patients cannot be visualized. The history and examination gives the examiner the correct answer.

There is no substitute for the one-on-one help a neurologist can give a patient with a chronic neurologic illness. The patient has someone to call, feels that this physician is knowledgeable about their illness and cares about them as a person. The physician can inspire the patient to keep trying and to realize that new discoveries occur daily. Most often, the patient inspires the neurologist by his or her courage and determination. Judgment of data and compassion for those who are ill will never be substituted by any form of imaging.

The fun of neurology is that you can make the diagnosis with your own brain and hands and now there is treatment. There has always been judgment and concern for those who are neurologically ill.

Index

CPSIA information can be obtained
at www.ICGtesting.com
Printed in the USA
BVHW021059190821
614776BV00019B/969